# GOD

*meets us in our*

*Suffering*

# GOD

*meets us in our*

# *Suffering*

HOPE AND ENCOURAGEMENT FOR THOSE
JOURNEYING THROUGH CANCER

## ROLF A. JACOBSON

*with* Karl N. Jacobson and Michael Pancoast

**Brazos Press**

*a division of Baker Publishing Group*
Grand Rapids, Michigan

Published by Brazos Press
a division of Baker Publishing Group
Grand Rapids, Michigan
BrazosPress.com

Printed in the United States of America

Library of Congress Cataloging-in-Publication Data
Names: Jacobson, Rolf A. author | Jacobson, Karl N., 1969– author | Pancoast, Michael author
Title: God meets us in our suffering : hope and encouragement for those journeying through cancer / Rolf A. Jacobson, with Karl N. Jacobson and Michael Pancoast.
Description: Grand Rapids, Michigan : Brazos Press, a division of Baker Publishing Group, [2026]
Identifiers: LCCN 2025025356 | ISBN 9781587436932 paperback | ISBN 9781493453757 ebook
Subjects: LCSH: Suffering—Religious aspects—Christianity | Hope—Religious aspects—Christianity | Cancer—Religious aspects—Christianity
Classification: LCC BV4909 .J256 2026 | DDC 248.8/6196994—dc23/eng/20250813
LC record available at https://lccn.loc.gov/2025025356

Stories told in this book reflect the authors' recollections of past experiences. Some names and characteristics have been changed, some events have been compressed, and some dialogue has been recreated.

Cover design by Christian Rafetto, Humble Books

Baker Publishing Group publications use paper produced from sustainable forestry practices and postconsumer waste whenever possible.

26  27  28  29  30  31  32        7  6  5  4  3  2  1

For all of the congregations
we have belonged to or served as pastors.
Especially for the pastors and people of
St. John's Lutheran Church (Northfield, MN)
Trinity Lutheran Church (Princeton, MN)
Lutheran Church of the Good Shepherd
(Minneapolis, MN)

And in memory of
Karl Nathaniel Jacobson
*Takk for alt*

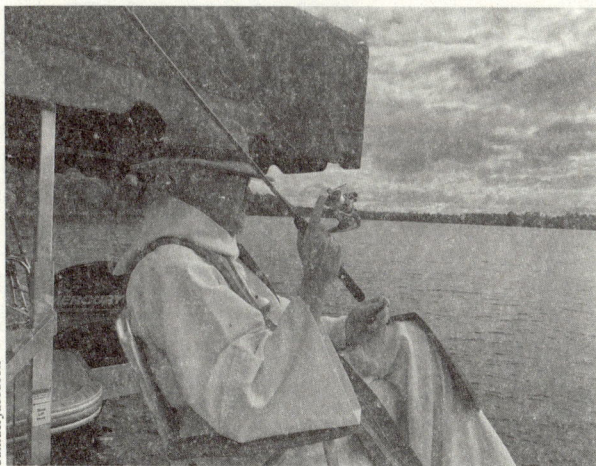

Samuel Jacobson

# CONTENTS

# PREFACE

This book was Karl's idea. It was Karl's idea that we three pastors—who had gone through cancer together—write a book about what it is like to go through a disease like cancer together. Along the way, as Mike and I (Rolf) weighed in, the book changed. It evolved dramatically in scope, organization, and direction. But it was Karl's idea.

I have been a cancer survivor since 1980. I had long insisted that I would never write a "cancer-memoir type of book." More than a few times, I was approached about the idea of writing such a book. But each time I declined, saying, "There are lots of books about cancer. The world doesn't need another one. It certainly doesn't need one from me."

But Karl wondered if there might not be a new angle. "This book starts with cancer, but it doesn't end there." This book will be different, he insisted, because it is about three people going through it together, because it will be written by three Christian pastors from the perspective of the "theology of the cross," and because it is really about life during and after illness. From that perspective, the truly important thing is that this book really isn't about cancer. It really isn't even about disease and disability. It is about life, faith, friendship, humor, loss, and hope.

Karl was right concerning what he imagined. In more ways than he knew. Here is what he wrote about the proposed book:

### This Book Isn't About Cancer . . . but It Starts There

All three of the authors of this book, Rolf, Mike, and Karl, have had cancer diagnoses. We know something about this disease. These diseases, we should say—after all, there are many different types of cancer. Cancer is not only the leading health crisis worldwide, it is also the leading cause of death worldwide. When it comes to cancer, there are all kinds of statistics: statistics about the various types of cancer; statistics having to do with age, gender, ethnicity; statistics about recovery and survival rates; statistics about recurrence; and even statistics about hair loss. Here is one pair of statistics to start with: As of 2023, 41 percent of men and 39 percent of women will be diagnosed with cancer at some point in their lifetime. This means that many of us will, at some point, be faced with such a diagnosis—either you or someone close to you will eventually be diagnosed with cancer. Odds are good—"good"?—odds *are* that cancer will come calling on you one way or another, in a diagnosis of your own or for someone close to you.

### When This Hard Reality Arises

First, a hard truth. Suffering is ugly and it is hard. Nobody wants to suffer, and most people do not want to look at suffering. Suffering—whether our own, that of those we care about, or even the suffering of complete strangers—is hard to endure and hard to stare in the face. Suffering scares us away for many reasons: because we don't know what to do, because we don't know how to help, because pain is frightening, because death and disability are terrifying, because all too often everything can seem beyond our power to change. We don't know what to say when someone is struggling with health (physical, emotional, spiritual, whatever), and in many cases there is literally nothing that we can do to make things better. And so, we turn away, not because we are bad people, but just the opposite.

Suffering is ugly. Suffering shows us our own helplessness. And a cancer diagnosis is the opening of a time of struggle and suffering; from surgery, to treatments that may halt or even kill cancer but often damage the body, to new realities in the aftermath of treatment, cancer means suffering. And this is not to mention all those other than the patient who are affected too—parents, spouses, children, and friends who struggle and suffer in their own right.

But suffering is also a place—the moment, the situation, the opportunity—where God can show up most powerfully, and where we can show up for each other too. And so . . .

## This Book Is About Faithfulness

This book is about faithfulness as the answer to cancer— God's faithfulness and ours. The three of us believe that our cancer stories are defined by faithfulness: the faithfulness that we believe God shows to us (to all of us); the hope and even joy that God's faithfulness evokes (even in the midst of suffering); the life-giving power of human faithfulness, one person to one another; and the gift of faithfulness as a refuge in times of trial.

What follows, then, is an invitation. An invitation to our stories as we have experienced the faithfulness of God in our own struggles. To the experiences that we have had of the faithfulness of family and friends. And to faithfulness as a concept that can help people make sense of life's darkest valleys, and show a way through them.

———

So what makes this book different? A few things.

The initial diagnosis for each of us was cancer—but it could have been some other illness, or some accident, or some other form of suffering. The book is really about the response to the initial diagnosis or suffering. It is about how God met us in our suffering, how we met each other, how we grew theologically and spiritually, how the church journeyed with us, and . . . well, there is another ending, as well. But that's for chapter 6.

This book is about three mutual perspectives on suffering. It is written by three people who went through cancer (and a lot of other tough stretches) together—side by side by side, as we like to say. This is not just one story, it is three. And it is not just one person's perspective, it is three people's perspectives.

This book is about the shared wisdom and spiritual truths that living with cancer and disability has afforded us. It is about *where* God meets us—in our suffering. It is also about *how* God meets us—in prayer, in giving and receiving care, in weakness, in the small kindnesses of tending our mutual humanity, of dreaming new dreams, and the like. The heart of the book—we hope—is in the spiritual reflection on our stories and engagement with the Bible on the questions our stories raise.

We also hope that this book is funny—at least, kind of funny . . . some of the time. When you look serious illness in the face, sometimes you just have to laugh. So we hope that at least some of the time this book is *ha-ha funny*. And some of the time it is *laugh-rather-than-cry funny* (if you know what we mean). And some of the time it is *ewwwww -icky funny*. And at the very end, we hope that the book is *Sarah-laughing-at-God funny* . . . or *Mary-laughing-because-Christ's-tomb-is-empty funny*. This book is about finding laughter in the midst of tears, joy in the midst of sorrow, beauty in the midst of ugliness, and love in the midst of . . . well, this book is just about love.

## "God Loves Raising People from the Dead"

Karl devoted almost all of 2022 and the first part of 2023 to his battle with cancer. He was able to return to ministry on Easter Sunday, April 9, 2023. During that sermon, he preached the following word of good news: "If there is one thing I've learned about the gospel in my time as a pastor, not to mention throughout my life—and if you'll bear with me, over the course of this past year my family and I have had—if there's one thing I've learned about the gospel, it's this: God loves raising people from the dead." In that "return from cancer" sermon, Karl named the most important thing that this book is about: life and death in the company of the God who raises the dead. One of the most important things the three of us have learned is how Christian congregations, at their best, are grace-filled communities where imperfect people take care of other imperfect people. Each of us experienced overwhelming love and care from many congregations of which we have been members—and especially from the congregations we belonged to when we each were diagnosed with cancer. So, we would like to dedicate this book to all of the congregations we have served or belonged to, and especially to the pastors and members of St. John's Lutheran Church, Northfield, Minnesota; Trinity Lutheran Church, Princeton, Minnesota; and the Lutheran Church of the Good Shepherd, Minneapolis, Minnesota. These are the congregations that the three of us belonged to when we were diagnosed. Thank you so much. And thank God for you.

When Karl pitched this book to me, he said, "This book will write itself." That was a nice sentiment, but, of course, books don't write themselves. Many people deserve thanks—they either contributed directly to this book or supported us as we worked on it. First, I want to thank Karl and Mike; writing a book with other people can test a person's patience. Since Karl and I have written together for many years, I was worried that we might drive Mike over the edge. He was patient, kind, diligent, and understanding—all of the things that he never usually is (just kidding, Mike). I also want to thank Karl's wife, Angela, for . . . everything. Words cannot express my appreciation—this is true also of Thursday, Sam, Lucy, Nora, and Claire. I am eager to thank my own wife, Amy, and our kids, Ingrid and Gunnar, for their constant support during this project. The year 2024 was not easy on any of us—we made it through together. On Mike's behalf, I also want to thank his wife Kari for her support along with their kids, Olsen, Laura, Anna, and Eleanor. My father, Del, gave Karl and me space and time at his cabin, where we wrote a major portion of this book; he listened to us and talked us through various parts of this project. Many people at Brazos Press earned our thanks through their customary excellent work, including Jim Kinney and James Korsmo. Thanks also to editor Amy Donaldson. As always, I wish to thank President Robin Steinke and the board of Luther Seminary for encouraging the faculty to publish scholarship for the church and for providing us with the support we need to do so. Thank you for the many ways in which you made this book possible. Thanks also to my partners in the academic dean's office—Terri, Jody, and Sandy—without whose teamwork and support this book would not have happened. And thanks for the many students, classmates, teachers, colleagues, friends, and relatives who have been part of our stories. Many of you show up in this book because you showed up in our lives. Thanks to Alan Padgett for reading early sections of this book and encouraging us.

A final note. As we narrate in chapter 6, Karl's health took a postcancer downturn, and he was not able to see this book to its completion. In a word, just after Karl was declared cancer free in the summer of 2024, he suddenly was struck down by another ailment—he was unconscious for a month and then he died. After Karl could no longer write, this book became for us a labor of love for Karl and also something of a tribute to him. Karl had written his sections in the first person, and much of it he wrote in the present tense. We believe Karl saw chapters 1–3 in close to a final form; chapters 4–5 had been started before Karl grew sick, although he didn't see very much of them; chapter 6 was written completely after his death. We chose to leave substantially "as is" everything that

Karl had written to that point. For chapter 6, we included some things that Karl had written in other places (such as sermons and blog posts) in order to get his voice into the chapter, but I narrate his story there.

As we complete the book, we therefore give thanks for Karl. The book of Proverbs contains this apt word of wisdom: "A friend loves at all times, and a brother is born to share adversity" (17:17; our translation). Karl and Mike were the closest of friends. Karl and Rolf were brothers who had also become friends. The three of us shared the adversity of cancer together, and we loved each other at all times. We give thanks to God for Karl's life, friendship, ministry, and witness to Jesus Christ. Karl, we love you and miss you more than the words in this book can ever express.

On behalf of Karl and Mike,
Rolf Jacobson
Christmas 2024—Mule Lake, Minnesota

# 1

# Diagnosis

## Dealing with the Disorienting News of Cancer

When I was well, I said to myself,
  "It won't happen to me."
By your grace, O LORD,
  you made me as healthy as a hill.
Then you hid your face;
  I was terrified.
        —Psalm 30:6–7 (our translation)

---

### ROLF (1980)

I was just coming out of what I was hoping was the worst part of my life—junior high. If you ever hope that you might experience reincarnation, just remember those two words—"junior high"—and realize that God doesn't reincarnate us because God is good. Our family had moved just before I started junior high, and those years weren't the greatest. But as I started tenth grade, I felt like I was finally getting established in the town of Northfield, Minnesota.

The previous summer, my sister Anne and I had biked on a four-day trip. Day 1: Northfield to Hudson, Wisconsin (about 60 miles, the way we went). Day 2: Hudson to Amery (about 45 miles). Day 3: Amery to River Falls (about 45 miles). Day 4: River Falls to Northfield (about 45 miles). We were supposed to make Northfield, anyway. But about 15 miles from home, I couldn't go any farther. My right leg hurt, and my stamina was gone.

A couple of weeks later, I went to tennis camp. The tennis part of the camp went pretty well. I played well, my game developed a great deal, and I was even awarded the Most Improved Player trophy. (In the words of Bill Murray's character in the movie *Stripes*, "Who could develop more than me? Talk about massive potential for growth!") In the mornings at camp, the students could go on a run with one of the counselors. I had never been fast, but I always had stamina. But I couldn't keep up with the other kids. By the end of the run, I was half a block behind. My stamina was gone.

End-of-summer chores around the house left me tired and in pain. My siblings thought I was lazy and a quitter, but the pain was real enough that I went to see our family doctor, Dr. Halvorson. Twice—once in August and again a month later. It turns out sarcoma—the type of cancer that was developing in my leg—is rare enough that most family physicians will never encounter a patient with it in their careers. And, as it turns out, it would have been impossible to detect even via a CT or bone scan at that point, even though I had symptoms.

2

Our doctor prescribed exercise. I was neither lazy nor a quitter, so I applied myself to exercise for over two months.

On Sunday, October 26, along with over thirty fellow tenth graders, I stood at the front of the sanctuary of St. John's Lutheran Church and confirmed my Christian faith. The Lutheran church teaches that God says yes to us in baptism. At confirmation, we say yes to God's yes. I still have a note that my godfather, Jim Limburg, wrote to me at my confirmation: "You've made a fine start on your life—we wish for you God's blessing in the years to come."

On Sunday, November 16, I was tossing the football in our front yard at halftime of the Vikings game. It was a peak-beautiful, fall day in Minnesota (you can look it up). The air was warm but dry. Dr. Halvorson lived next door and was gardening in his yard. My dad called him over to look at my leg, which was still bothering me. He took one look at my femur, which now had significant swelling, and said with alarm, "It didn't look like this before. Come see me again tomorrow." After the game, my parents went out for dinner. The Vikings beat Tampa Bay 38–30 (you can look it up).

I was home alone when Dr. Halvorson knocked on our door a couple of hours later, asking for my parents. I told him they were out for dinner in the Twin Cities with my aunts and an uncle. He said, "Get in my car. We are going to the hospital. I want to get an X-ray of your leg."

It was a different world in 1980. Parents would let a nineteen-year-old girl and her fifteen-year-old brother go on a four-day bike trip by themselves. Doctors could have a kid X-rayed without the consent of either his parents or the insurance company—as I remember, Dr. Halvorson operated the X-ray by himself.

3

My parents returned home around midnight. Dr. Halvorson had been watching for them and was knocking on our door before they even sat down. My parents got me out of bed. Holding up an X-ray over a living room lamp, Dr. Halvorson explained that I might have a tumor in my leg. He had called the Mayo Clinic in Rochester, Minnesota. They were expecting us first thing in the morning.

By the end of a day of medical tests on Monday, I was exhausted. My stamina was gone to the point that I could barely stand in the elevator. Late in the afternoon, I met Dr. Frank Sim for the first time. He walked into the little consulting room on the fourteenth floor of Mayo, followed by a small army of medical students, residents, and visiting surgeons from around the world. After making introductions, he jammed an X-ray into the light screen and pointed. I'll never forget his words. "We have a problem. This is cancer. Tomorrow, we will check him into the hospital. First thing Wednesday morning, we will amputate his leg and this boy will live a normal life." I can still hear the ringing silence that ensued. (He clearly didn't know me; if he did, he would never have said that I would live a normal life.)

More discussion followed, led by my dad. My dad will tell you that I hated it a little bit when he asked doctors questions. He is wrong. I *hated it a lot* when he asked doctors questions, even if they were good questions. What kind of cancer do you think it is? *Osteosarcoma (bone cancer)*. Why amputate, why not just cut the tumor out? *It doesn't work*. What caused this cancer? *We don't know*. And so on.

We were sent to see the oncologists next. Oncologists—aka, doctors with feelings. They explained that surgeons weren't always right. There was a chance that it wasn't cancer.

Even if it was cancer, there was some good news. There was no sign of cancer anywhere else in my body, especially in my lungs, which is where osteosarcoma spreads. So there was no need for chemotherapy at the moment. (Spoiler alert: The cancer had already spread to my lungs. The dozens of tiny tumors in each lung simply weren't large enough for a Jimmy Carter–era CT scan to detect yet.) They sent in the social worker next—Carol.

On Wednesday, November 19, they amputated my right leg above the knee. The last thing I remember of that day was lying on a gurney, waiting to be wheeled into surgery, visiting with a fellow who was also awaiting surgery. When they came to get me, he said, "May God bless you."

And you know what? God has indeed blessed me. The whirlwind diagnosis and amputation were a staggering blow. The discovery the following April that the cancer had spread to my lungs was a further blow (more on that in a later chapter). But the innumerable blessings that flowed my way through so many people in the months and years since then have been mind-blowing. Those blessings have come through so many people. My immediate family and my (almost) innumerable extended family. Our church—especially the members of American Lutheran Church Women of St. John's Lutheran Church. My teachers and coaches. My musical mates. My friends and my friends' parents. (Shortly before my mom died, someone asked me what was the key to winning my war with cancer. My mom piped up, "Great friends!") Our neighbors and the wonderful love of many townsfolk in Northfield, Minnesota.

---

## MIKE (2022)

On Friday, January 14, 2022, I was doing what every pastor I've ever known absolutely *loves* doing: a high school youth lock-in. Not surprisingly, over the course of that evening I experienced some stomach discomfort—who wouldn't experience some "stomach discomfort" after an evening of pizza, chips, pop, and other youth favorites?! So, I paid it no mind.

As the evening wound down, I retired to my pallet rolled out in a corner of the church's fellowship hall, knowing that, whether the kids slept or not, I was in for a long night. For the past two weeks, since my wife Kari and I and our young adult children had spent the Christmas holiday with her family at her folks' lake place outside Aitkin, Minnesota, I had been experiencing some lower-back pain. But I had dismissed that pain. I attributed it to sleeping on a middling mattress, rather than the lovely mattress we have at home. So, *both* the stomach and back discomfort that evening at the church were not promising factors for a good night's sleep, never mind whatever hijinks the youth had up their sleeves. But again, I paid that back pain no mind. (Detecting a pattern here?)

The next morning, I cooked breakfast for the youth to wrap up the event, helped with cleanup, and spent a couple of hours in my office to prepare for the next day's Sunday service, before heading home. By the time I returned home, the night's stomach discomfort had morphed into occasional waves of sharp pain. Darn kids and their junk food. But as the evening wore on, the pain increased, and each wave increasingly sharpened, enough that by supper time I had to admit to Kari: "I think I'm going to have to have you get me to the emergency room." As we headed to the car, I experienced a wave of abdominal pain like I had never encountered before. It dropped me to my knees and took my breath away. There was no room for not paying any mind to this.

After I checked in at the ER, a bout of diarrhea seemed to relieve the pain—darn kids and their junk food. But, since we were there, at Kari's insistence (I was ready to go home) "we" decided it was best to get this checked out. The ER doctor began to examine me for what he thought could be possible culprits: gallbladder, appendix, kidney stones. Nothing in my blood or urine labs indicated any of these. And, since the pain had subsided, I was discharged with the advice to check back in with our primary care provider.

Which was fortuitous. Unbeknownst to Kari, I had already scheduled an appointment for later that week. Since around Thanksgiving, I had noticed a small lump on the right side of my neck. I had been battling cold symptoms (but not COVID-19) off and on throughout the fall. I thought the lump must just be an inflamed lymph node like anyone might have when one's body is battling an illness. Little did I know I was only partially right. But with the Advent and Christmas seasons looming, I paid that little lump no mind. (Yeah, definitely a pattern.) But since the lump never went away and seemed also to grow some, I thought it best, without saying anything to my spouse, to make an appointment to have it checked.

On Thursday, January 20, 2022, I went in for that appointment. Our physician's assistant felt my neck. She pressed on my abdomen and back. Looking at my blood and urine labs, she had some pointed questions about family health history, with one question in particular bringing me up short: Any occurrence of lymphoma or other blood-related cancers? My sister Kristen is a Hodgkin's lymphoma survivor. (Turns out, there is no family-history correlation at all between Hodgkin's and non-Hodgkin's lymphoma—I was simply about to "win the lottery.") But in my health-care provider's mind, the things to which I had paid no mind were all related. So, an ultrasound was scheduled for that very day for both my abdomen and neck, with a follow-up appointment scheduled for Friday to read the results. The ultrasound revealed enlarged lymph nodes in my neck, chest, and abdomen. The latter, being in very close proximity with my right kidney, were the likely culprit of what I was reporting as "back pain."

The next-day follow-up with our physician's assistant led to a recommendation for a CT scan with contrast dye just to find out the extent of these swollen lymph nodes. That appointment came the following Monday, January 24—we were fully a week into this sudden and strange ordeal.

Beginning with that CT scan, I had to learn to deal with the embarrassment that was part and parcel of some of the procedures. I had to learn to either laugh or cry—so I did my best to laugh. The CT tech told me that when the dye was administered, I would begin to feel an "unusual warmth" that would begin at my shoulders and progress through the rest of my body, ending in my "groin and behind area." What the tech didn't tell me is that there were two *very specific* areas in my groin and behind—a little nugget of knowledge over which Karl and I were later able to share a laugh!

Before I had even returned home, I had the results of that scan on my handheld device that doubles as a phone, results not wrapped in medical speak: "suspected lymphoma" located (or "diffused") throughout my neck, chest, and lower abdomen. The next procedure would be an ultrasound-guided needle biopsy to tap into one of the swollen nodes, which would tell us much more about what we were dealing with.

With all this news, information, and questions swirling, I was given an opportunity from two of my most trusted friends and confidants, Karl and Rolf, to join them and their dad, Del, for a couple of days of good food and drink at Del's cabin on Mule Lake near Longville, Minnesota. The needle biopsy had not been scheduled yet, and there was a good chance the call could come while I was at the cabin. After a couple of days with my pals, sure enough, the call came: biopsy scheduled for Thursday, January 27. The biopsy revealed, indeed, stage 3, diffuse large B-cell non-Hodgkin's lymphoma.

The only other wrinkle in this part of the saga was, it turns out, there is no such thing as "just" non-Hodgkin's lymphoma. The next step was to determine the genetic labeling of my lymphoma, not only to determine its particular flavor, but more importantly to figure out what treatment offered the best response. That was when I met Dr. Hani Alkhatib, an oncologist with CentraCare based out of St. Cloud, Minnesota: "We will be treating you not just for remission—which is our first goal—but for a cure." That was on Monday, February 7. "It takes us a while to do that genetic tagging," he concluded.

Unfortunately, or fortunately—I'm not even sure if either of those words is appropriate—on Wednesday, February 9, I encountered another bout of that abdominal/lower-back pain that first put me on this journey, this time worse than before! A second of what would become numerous trips to the ER ensued. It was suspected that my swollen lymph nodes were even more swollen, pressing on things not normally pressed, and causing me all this pain. A bed space was procured at the St. Cloud hospital, and without the genetic tagging in hand, Dr. Alkhatib, thankfully, ordered the start of my first round of chemotherapy, a cocktail called R-CHOP: rituximab, Cytoxan, hydroxydaunomycin (doxorubicin hydrochloride or Adriamycin, affectionately called "the red devil"), Oncovin (vincristine), and super-high doses of prednisone. Dr. Alkhatib was confident this initial round of chemo would immediately shrink my lymph nodes and bring relief, and once the genetic tagging came back, we would know if we needed to change cocktails. He was right. On Friday, February 11, I was discharged from my first round of chemo pain free and with the lump in my neck almost gone.

On Thursday, February 17, I returned to the Coborn Cancer Clinic for a follow-up with Dr. Alkhatib. The genetic tagging indicated my flavor of lymphoma required a more targeted version of chemo going forward, a cocktail called R-EPOCH—same as R-CHOP but with an additional drug in the cocktail, plus a chaser called methotrexate, which crosses into one's spinal cord to make sure there aren't any rogue cancer cells camped out there. Recurrence, if/when it occurs, often shows up in the spinal cord or brain.

Thus began what would become five five-day in-hospital R-EPOCH treatments and three more three-day in-hospital treatments of methotrexate (interrupted once by a weeklong COVID bout, just for fun).

Through it all, I encountered—even in my suffering, or perhaps because I was suffering—the presence of God through Christ Jesus. Martin Luther used to say that in Holy Communion the body of Jesus Christ is mysteriously present "in, with, and under" the bread and the wine.[1] At the lowest point of my cancer and chemotherapy, I experienced Christ as present in, with, and under the suffering—I *encountered Jesus* there. This encounter occurred through the efforts, well-wishes, cards, meals, phone calls, and visits from my family. Through the congregation I was serving at the time, Trinity Lutheran Church in Princeton, Minnesota. Through my friends. Through the medical staff associated with the CentraCare system. God promises to meet us in the cross, in suffering. Because of my experience of Christ's presence in the very part of my life when it felt like God was not going to be present, but was, this has meant for me an expansion of my faith's imagination to be apprehended by and met by God, through faith, in these other ways by my family, my friends, and more.

---

## KARL (2022)

To paraphrase our mutual friend Hans, "2022 can go straight to hell." It was Wednesday, February 16, 2022—three weeks after Mike's biopsy. When we'd been together at my dad's lake place and I'd complained about some back pain of my own, Mike's unspoken thought at the time was, "Oh no, he's got it too."

I'd been having back and chest pain for a while. I'd had one virtual visit with a doctor, which ruled out heart issues (this entailed lots of going up and down stairs at home, getting the heart rate up, and so on, which my dog loved supervising). I had a follow-up appointment scheduled for an in-person visit on Thursday afternoon. That Wednesday night I had the worst night of sleep I'd ever had: pain, shaking, and vomiting

11

(due, my doctor later told me, to the pain in my back). My wife, Angela, was on sabbatical at a remote mountain retreat in the Cascade Mountains of Washington, and I had our three daughters at home. Thursday morning, I asked my stepdaughter Nora (the only other driver in the house) to get her sister Claire and her stepsister Lucy to school so that I could go to urgent care right away. I said that I'd see them later in the afternoon. I didn't get home for a month.

After some blood work at the urgent care, they sent me to the ER at Regions Hospital in St. Paul but told me that I couldn't drive myself, since I apparently had neither blood pressure nor white blood cells. I called my brother Rolf, who lived and worked nearby, and he drove me to the ER. By noon, I'd had a bone marrow biopsy, and I'd received an initial diagnosis of leukemia. They said, "We suspect you have leukemia." I asked, looking for clarification, "So, you're going to test for leukemia?" Rolf answered for the doctor (Rolf will answer for anybody), "Karl, they're telling you that you have leukemia."

Toward the end of the day, Rolf asked a doctor, "Is Karl staying here tonight?" The doctor replied, "He isn't leaving here for a month!"

The general diagnosis was expanded to B-cell acute lymphoblastic leukemia (ALL), with the added bonus of being positive for the Philadelphia chromosome—a genetic mutation due to which parts of two chromosomes (numbers 9 and 22) break off and switch places, before reattaching. Philadelphia "positive." Right. "City of brotherly love." Uh-huh. I'm still not over the Vikings versus Eagles 2018 NFC title game. Words like "Philadelphia" and "positive" could go the way of 2022.

The goal was to treat to "first remission," killing as much of the leukemia as possible, after which a bone marrow transplant (BMT) would be the only path to a cure. A transplant is not done unless the cancer count is less than 5 percent of one's blood cells. As my doctor said, "You gotta be below five. Four would be okay. Three would be better. One would be better still. What we'd really like is zero, 'cause zero is best." (Zero percent cancer is better than 5 percent? Really?! Shocking what medical school will teach you.) So, treatment was chemotherapy, which included spinal taps (now more often called "lumbar punctures," because that's less scary, and less B movie) to introduce chemo medication into the spinal fluid prophylactically in order to prevent the leukemia from settling in the spine and brain. All of this took place over the course of three months, some inpatient, some outpatient.

After the first round of treatment, I was in line for a clinical trial, something called CAR-T treatment, which is an immunotherapy that teaches one's T cells (lymphocytic cells that fight infections/disease) to bind to cancer cells and kill them. This would reduce my "residual disease" to as close to absolute zero as possible, in preparation for the BMT.

But blood work in preparation for the trial showed that the flavor of leukemia I had wasn't actually ALL, but CML—chronic myeloid leukemia. How could that be? Was it a secondary cancer? Was it a misdiagnosis? No, as it turns out, it was a change. As it happens, ALL can, sometimes, in very rare cases, transform into CML. This happens in about 1 percent of all ALL cases, which made me, as one of my nurses said, "A real unicorn." She had never seen this in more than twenty years at the BMT clinic.

While I remained in the first-remission stage, my cells were in what is called "lymphoid blast crisis"—basically meaning they were about to go turbo, which is usually fatal. So, we were back on board the transplant train, ASAP (lots of abbreviations are explained here, but you already know that one).

I've compared this experience to a roller coaster, while Angela has called it whiplash. (You can get whiplash on a roller coaster, by the way, so we're both right.) After further chemo treatments and four radiation treatments to kill my bone marrow and make room for new marrow, I was ready for the BMT. Both of my sisters were a match to be my donor, but the doctor chose firstborn sister Anne. Proving that it doesn't always pay to be older.

On June 14, 2022, I had a bone marrow transplant composed of five hundred million bone marrow cells. Five hundred million, which at the time reminded me of comedian Mitch Hedberg's joke about rice: "Rice is great when you're hungry, and you want two thousand of something." Five hundred million bone marrow cells, which meant a chance at second remission, and potentially a cure.

But the reality is that there were and are more statistics. There is 20–25 percent mortality rate because of the transplant procedure alone. This is then followed by the risk of what is called "graft versus host disease." Every kind of transplant—organ, tissue, and so on—runs the risk of rejection. Typically, it is the body that rejects the new organ or graft, but when it comes to bone marrow, the risk is for the graft bone marrow to reject the host body. It's kind of like when you throw a party when your parents are out of town, and some of your rowdy friends who come to the kegger go, "Hey, wait a minute, this isn't our house, let's trash the place."

I spent thirty days in the hospital, followed by seventy more days at home, during which I couldn't be left alone and had to be within thirty minutes of the clinic, in case I experienced graft versus host disease. I survived the transplant and, like FDR (here I'm talking about the president; all these abbreviations are great, aren't they?), my first one hundred days were a success.

One year later, in June of 2023, a bone marrow biopsy showed no sign of disease—of either cancer or genetic mutation. My physical recovery was slow. I still have fatigue, weakness, and days where I have no energy at all, and from what I gather, I will likely never be at 100 percent again. All along there have been troubling numbers, statistics, and odds that have been in front of me. One of five BMT patients does not survive; three in five recover with significant limitations. There is something like a 40–45 percent recurrence rate even after transplant. But, as the great Han Solo said in *The Empire Strikes Back*, "Never tell me the odds!"

What got me to this point, through a difficult passage and ready to face what might come next, is that I was strangely well prepared for all of this. I had a family of origin shaped by faith. I watched my parents navigate my brother's cancer, how they dealt with what it all meant for our whole family. I've had my brother as an example of how to face cancer and life after cancer with courage and humor. I have phenomenal friends, generous members of the congregation I was pastoring at the time, supportive family members, and a partner in my wife Angela, who was (and is) remarkable. And, being able to walk with Mike, "side by side" through cancer, as we've said from the beginning, has made all the difference in the world. (Although as Mike's wife Kari said, "You guys need to find something better to do 'side by side.'")

But Mike and I have been using the language of "side by side" for a good while now, because our diagnoses were so close together, and we've been doing things side by side for almost thirty years—from our time as classmates at Luther Seminary, to marriages, children, callings, continuing education, and more. And for each of us, at numerous times in our lives, and indeed all along, there have been others who stood by our side. This is, we firmly believe, the key to facing anything, everything, that life might throw at us—the bad and the good—sticking side by side, by side, by side, by side. In other words, faithfulness.

And, of course, according to Psalm 23, when facing any crisis—cancer, illness, divorce, unemployment, aging, death—God is the faithful Good Shepherd who walks side by side with those who enter the valley of the shadow of death. As the King James Version puts it, "Yea, though I walk through the valley of the shadow of death, I will fear no evil: for thou art with me." And according to Psalm 23 and the other psalms of trust,[2] God is present with sufferers not merely in an intellectual or emotional sense. Rather, God is with sufferers in spiritually powerful ways. Psalm 23 describes God's presence as similar to a shepherd's rod and staff: "Your rod and your staff comfort me." The rod and staff were the shepherd's tools to fend off predators and also to keep the sheep in line. God is similarly present with sufferers in powerful ways—bringing sufferers through crisis and into a new day.

## The Immediate Aftermath of a Shattering Diagnosis or Disastrous News

A cancer diagnosis can be a shock—especially when it comes out of nowhere to punch a seemingly healthy person right in the face. It can be shattering. This can be true of any significant, sudden trauma: a heart attack, the sudden death of a loved one, a major accident, the unexpected loss of a job, being the victim of a crime, and so on. One day, Rolf was a fairly typical tenth grader. A couple of days later he only had one leg. What do you do with a closet full of tennis, ski, and marching band gear? One morning, Karl was rebuilding his life with a new wife and a new job. By the end of that day, he was confined to a cancer ward for a month. How do you respond when the wind is taken out of your sails so suddenly? One month, Mike was doing his best to fight through chronic pain in order to lead a congregation and father a family. Then, suddenly, he was forced to focus his energy on his own body . . . which was trying to kill him. What next?

Being diagnosed with a severe illness can be shattering. So can other disastrous news, such as the sudden death of a loved one, being fired from a wonderful job, being told by one's spouse that they are divorcing you, and the like. We simply want to acknowledge how devastating bad news can be. As individuals, the three of us have received such shocking news more than a few times. Many more times, as pastors, we have journeyed with others who have been greeted with similarly crushing news; the examples are too numerous and painful to list.

The very first challenge is simply to absorb the news. Bad news can be like a winter gust of twenty-degree-below-zero blizzard. You're just overwhelmed. You literally struggle to understand the words. Someone says, "You have cancer." Or, "I regret to inform you that your spouse is dead." And you think, "What? Can you say that again? I don't understand." Sometimes, when you immerse a really large, old sponge in water, it takes a while for the sponge to absorb the water—it isn't instantaneous. And you can't rush the process. The first challenge is to give yourself *and your loved ones* the space to absorb the news. In September 2020, Rolf was awakened one morning by a text from our friend Hans's wife saying that Hans had had a stroke. Rolf had to read the text three times before it could make sense. Then he had to wake his wife Amy and read it to her three times before she could wrap her brain around it. Some thinkers embrace the old "cycle of grief" model, which describes the process as including things such as denial, anger, bargaining, depression, and acceptance. (Our friend Hans jokingly proposes other stages such as "pro-crastination," "doom scrolling," and "fully body itch.") Not everyone goes through each of these stages, but the stages do help to name the difficulty of letting the crushing news soak in. In the Bible, after Job lost all of his property, all of his kids, and then his health, he is pictured as sitting in the ashen ruins of his life. Eugene Peterson offers a gut-wrenching paraphrase of the scene: "Job was ulcers and scabs from head to foot. They itched and oozed so badly that he took a piece of broken pottery to scrape himself, then went and sat on a trash heap, among the ashes" (Job 2:7–8 The Message). Though the scene is heartrending, it does offer a poignant image of what it is like to receive devasting news.

So what do you do when you suddenly find yourself sitting in the ashes of your shattered life? As we've already said, the first step is to let the news soak in. And don't rush that part. And, of course, as pastors we encourage everyone to seek God as best you (or your faith community) are able to do so. Call a pastor! Even if you haven't been to church in forty years, call a pastor. More on seeking God later in this book. As we reflect on the beginnings of our battles with cancer, we offer three other thoughts in this chapter: (1) the power of denial and learning *to pay attention* to one's body; (2) the *importance of slowing down to care for your health* and admitting that you can't do everything yourself; and (3) the reality that medical care can dehumanize a person, so one must *tend what is human* in a person.

## The Power of Denial and Learning to Pay Attention to One's Body

For reasons that are both similar and dissimilar, Mike and Rolf waited too long to get the proper medical attention and diagnosis. Here is a truth about human nature: We are not good at receiving bad news. When we get bad news or even think bad news might be coming, we often choose to ignore it, and at times some people actively choose to believe something other than reality. This fact about human nature is so true that even when there is overwhelming evidence that something is not right, we still often choose not to face it head-on. It's called *denial*. Denial is not just for those struggling with chemical dependency who aren't ready to face reality. Denial can be a reaction to any life-altering news, such as the signs of or diagnosis of a disease.

There is another problematic aspect of human nature that, when combined with denial, can multiply one's problems.

19

One might call this pride, fear of embarrassment, aversion to asking for help, or other names. In 1980, Rolf experienced enough pain and exhaustion that he went to the doctor twice. After the second visit, he didn't want to go back a third time because of fear of embarrassment. Rolf was afraid the doctor and others would think he was the boy who cried wolf (which is kind of funny, because the name Rolf means "wolf"). Twice the doctor had examined him and prescribed exercise. In the two months that followed, the tumor grew slowly, but it grew to the point that the swelling was noticeable. Rolf should have returned to the doctor, but pride and fear of embarrassment kept him away. Only the fortuitous fact that his family physician lived next door allowed the cancer to be diagnosed when it was. Mike's story is similar—he ignored symptoms such as a lump on his neck, pain in his back, stomach discomfort, drop-you-to-your-knees abdominal pain, and finally diarrhea. Even at the ER, once the diarrhea relieved this stomach pain, he was ready to return home. Only the fortuitous wisdom of his wife, Kari, kept him there long enough to get examined. Why? Oh, let's guess—pride, denial, fear of embarrassment. And for both Rolf and Mike, the inconvenient truth that our society tells men that bearing pain is manly. "Don't worry, I can handle the pain. Just throw me that bottle of aspirin."

The power of denial, pride, and fear of embarrassment is not just a psychological or emotional problem; *it is a spiritual problem*. And spiritual problems demand spiritual responses. The book of Proverbs says, "Before a disaster, there is pride; and before a fall, there is a haughty spirit" (16:18; our translation). Pride and fear of embarrassment can stem from overconfidence ("I can handle it" or "I can bear the pain") or insecurity ("I might be embarrassed" or "They might think I'm weak").

### The Importance of Slowing Down to Care for Your Health

Another major factor in human nature that often prevents people from getting timely diagnosis and treatment is busyness. People who are too busy—or who are too focused on all of the tasks in front of them—often fail to attend to basic life matters, such as health or helping someone. In his book *The Tipping Point*, Malcolm Gladwell made famous the results of an experiment that two Princeton University researchers, by the name of Darley and Batson, conducted in 1973 with some Princeton Theological Seminary students. The experiment was inspired by a parable of Jesus, in which a man was beaten, robbed, and left for dead on a road (Luke 10:29–37). In Jesus's parable, a Levite and a priest pass by the man and don't help him; but a third traveler—a Samaritan—helps the man. Gladwell writes that the seminary students were asked to prepare a short speech—a sermon—on this parable. Then they were sent to another building to deliver the speech. Some students were told they needed to hurry, because they were late. Other students were told that they could take their time. Along the way to the next building, the researchers had placed a man slumped in an alley, as if beaten and robbed. The researchers wondered which of these aspiring ministers—having just prepared a message about three men who encountered a beaten-and-robbed man—would stop to help. The answer? About 10 percent of the students who were told that they were late stopped to help. But over 60 percent of those who were told that they had plenty of time to get to the next building stopped to offer help. Gladwell concluded, "The words 'Oh, you're late' had the effect of making someone who was ordinarily compassionate into someone who was indifferent to suffering—of turning someone, in that particular moment, into a different person."[3] For our purposes in this book, the point is that those who are too busy are more likely to fail to care for themselves and for others. When we are consumed with all of the *things* we need to get done, we are less likely to care for *people—including ourselves.*

There is again a spiritual element to the problem of being overly busy. There is a temptation to think, "If I don't do it, nobody will do it, or worse—they will do it wrong." Or, "If I don't show up, maybe people will realize that they don't need me." Or, "If I don't get this deal, I won't have enough—enough money, enough success, or enough influence." At the heart of this focus on the next meeting or task is the sin of putting ourselves at the center of our own universe. We become the star of our own drama and the narrator of our own story. It is a form of idolatry—worshiping something other than the one, true God. Placing something other than God at the center of our lives. God is the center of existence—the creator of all, the savior of all, the Lord who loves and guides all.

In Martin Luther's Large Catechism, in his explanation of the first commandment—"You shall have no other gods before me"—he wrote, "A god is that to which we look for all good and in which we find refuge in every time of need."[4] When we become workaholics—or get so busy that we cannot tend to our health—we are functionally becoming our own gods. We become the thing we worship; we become our

22

own false gods. The thing about worshiping a false god rather than the true God is that false gods don't keep promises. False gods are not capable of bearing the weight of our worship. They are not able to rescue us from distress or crisis.

God's answer to our broken tendency to place ourselves at the center of our own drama and to get lost in busyness is the Sabbath. The word "sabbath" (Hebrew *shabbat*) literally means "stop." Stop working so hard. Your body and your spirit need rest. Taking a full day off from work won't make you go broke—you will have enough. And taking a day off will give your mind time to attend to the things that you are neglecting when you lose yourself in your busyness. A farmer we know refused to work on Sundays. He said, "If I can't make this farm profitable working six days a week, something is wrong!" He was right—and not just about himself, but about all of us.

In the Bible, the sabbath isn't just one day a week—it is also a general principle that calls for regular rest. The sabbath principle calls for people to rest one day in seven, for the land to rest one year in seven, for debts to be forgiven one year in seven, for slaves to go free after seven years, and for all land to be returned to the original family owners one year in every forty-nine (seven times seven years). The sabbath principle extends logically to worship—worship the Lord every seventh day, but also worship the Lord for major festivals three times a year. Logically, it also implies time with God every day and a period of rest and quiet every day.

Such regular periods of resting and stopping all the busyness—on a daily basis, on a weekly basis, on an annual basis, on an every-seven-years basis—allow a person to listen to God and to listen to their own body. Or, in Mike's case, to listen to one's wife, so that one can get the medical treatment that is needed.

Such stopping, listening, and obeying one's wife requires humility. It means asking for help. It means admitting that one's presence or activity is not as indispensable as one had thought. Humility is really hard. Asking for and receiving help is really hard. But sometimes a little humility—even if it is hard—can save your life. Humility is essential when battling illness or any trauma.

Here is an urgent word of advice for newly diagnosed people (or their caregivers). *Be your own advocate!* One piece of advice that we give to everyone who is diagnosed with cancer is *to be your own most assertive advocate.* Medical systems can be slow. (If time were raindrops, Mike could fill up many a rain barrel with the hours he spent trying to get various treatments authorized by his insurance provider.) As a patient or a caregiver, with as much humility and urgency as you can gather, press for the care that you want. Do not be afraid to tell your providers how you are feeling and what you think you need. And that includes God. As an old gospel tune says, "Call him up, call him up, *tell him what you want.*"

## Medical Care Dehumanizes, So Tend What Is Human in a Person

Earlier Mike mentioned his encounter with the CT scan tech's polite, genteel description of the warm feeling from the contrast dye in his "groin and behind area." The reality of that experience was a not-so-unpleasant feeling, specifically in his penis (Can we write "penis" in a book like this?!) and anus (Can we write "anus" in a book like this?!), like an ever so tender "poof." That realization was cathartically humorous enough, literally eliciting a little giggle right there on the CT scan bed. But later, when Mike found out Karl, too, would be having a CT scan, Mike told Karl: "Okay. They're likely going to tell you about the warm feeling starting with your shoulders and ending in your groin and behind area. It's waaaaay more specific than that!" It wasn't just funny to share that with Karl then. It continued to be funny when Karl later confirmed, "So *that's* what you meant!"

One of the things to know about severe illness is that medical care can dehumanize a person. Medical care can diminish a person's humanity, either by making a person feel less human or by literally taking away a part of their humanity. A friend of mine reminded me of a poignant line from Jason Isbell's song "Elephant," sung from the perspective of "Andy," whose lover is dying of cancer. "One thing that's real clear to me: no one dies with dignity. We just try to ignore the elephant somehow." The "elephant" is both death and the dehumanizing way cancer kills. At the most basic level, this dehumanizing can occur when medical professionals treat the disease rather than care for the person with the disease. Almost all medical professionals know this and make extreme goodwill efforts to care for the person with the disease, rather than just fight the disease. But it is almost inevitable that when a person has a long-term fight with a disease, they will at some point feel like the physicians are treating the disease more than the person.

This potentially dehumanizing aspect of medical care starts with low-grade interactions. The patient is poked, prodded, and palpitated. The patient is stabbed with needles, scanned with X-rays, and penetrated in other uncomfortable ways. The patient is required to strip naked in front of strangers. The patient may be cut with scalpels, burned with radiation, or poisoned with chemotherapy. (One of Rolf's oncologists said, "We only know three ways to treat this disease: cut, burn, and poison.") In Rolf's case, part of his humanity was cut off: his legs. In Karl's case, part of his humanity was killed by chemotherapy and radiation: his bone marrow. In Mike's case, he never had a human soul, so there was nothing to dehumanize.

In Karl's case . . . yeah, his case was super special. He mentioned four radiation treatments. Actually, there were six: the four full-body treatments and two extra-special, targeted treatments. Leukemia isn't like other cancers, in that there aren't "stages." Leukemia doesn't start as a tumor and then metastasize, spreading to other parts of the body, as was the case with Rolf's cancer, or with Mike's diagnosis of "diffuse" (i.e., spread) large B-cell non-Hodgkin's lymphoma. Leukemia is already running all through you. It can, however, "hide." And where does it hide? Two places. One is the brain, so his fifth radiation treatment targeted his brain—which, after they found his brain, went smoothly enough. The second place leukemia can hide is . . . um . . . well, may we leave it at "lower"? Further south? Is this making you, dear reader, as uncomfortable as it is me? Okay, out with it, using the technical medical term: the testicles. And let us tell you, that process wasn't nearly as smooth as the brain blast. It took three University of Minnesota medical residents to set it up (two young women and one young man, all three half Karl's age). Here, we will let Karl speak for himself:

> There I was, lying on my back, while they taped my penis
> (We agreed we would use technical medical terms, right?)

26

to my stomach, and put a half-inch-thick lead plate between my testicles, and radiated my testicles for fifteen minutes from each side. I've never felt so exposed, so vulnerable, and so humiliatingly on display in all my life. And as I lay there, my mind racing with embarrassed, nerve-racking energy, I kept saying to myself, "I am as God made me! I am as God made me!" To add insult to injury, after it was over the doctor informed me that the radiation treatment would "eliminate any possibility of impregnation." So, I guess all that money I spent on that vasectomy was wasted.

If medical care can be dehumanizing, what is the answer? *You tend what is human in the patient.* Tend what is human! According to Genesis 1:26–28, every human is created in the image of God. You tend what is human in a person by cultivating and nurturing that divine image in a person—their creativity, their growth and development, their hopes and dreams, their passions, their ability to love and be loved, their sense of humor. This is what Jerry Seinfeld meant when he said, "Humor is the most powerful, most survival-essential quality you will ever have or need to navigate through the human experience."[5] For "humor," in that sentence, one might substitute music, art, literature, sports, food, games, adventure, friendship, and many other worthy aspects of the human experience. This can, of course, be a problem if the disease or accident takes away a person's passion, as it did with Rolf. Rolf had loved playing tennis and being in the marching band. Those were taken away suddenly. So other passions needed to be nurtured in their place—guitar, reading, puzzles, friendship. A different and new part of humanity sometimes has to be nurtured.

If you are the patient, tend what is human in yourself. Reread a favorite book. Listen to your favorite music. Take time on nice days to sit outside and literally smell the flowers. Go hunting, fishing, or bird-watching. Call a long-lost friend. Get a massage. Go out for dinner and order a Grand Marnier. Get another massage. You are human; tend what is human in yourself.

If you are a caregiver, tend what is human in the one you love or care for. If they're confined to bed, wash their hair or hold their hand. Bring a book of pictures from their childhood and ask questions about the photos. Let them win at *Settlers of Catan*. Watch a baseball game or a favorite movie. They are human; tend what is human in them.

Also, if you are a caregiver, tend what is human in yourself. And care for your own health. Oh, and slow down. Caregivers often take on too much and experience a decline in their own health and sense of well-being. So apply all of these things to yourself, if you're a caregiver. Tend what is human in yourself.

If you are a friend, walk with the patient side by side, as we have done. Or rather, side by side by side. And if you are a dog, well, you are probably the best tender of humanity that a patient can have, so be yourself. Because who knows how to tend what is human in a human better than a dog? I suppose you want a treat now.

# 2

# Treatment

## When God Shows Up in Your Suffering

Out of the depths I cry to you, O LORD.
  Lord, hear my voice! . . .
I wait for the LORD, my soul waits,
  and in his word I hope;
my soul waits for the Lord
  more than those who watch for the morning,
  more than those who watch for the morning.
  —Psalm 130:1–2a, 5–6

---

### ROLF (1981)

After my initial cancer diagnosis and leg amputation in 1980, there was no sign of the disease elsewhere in my body. Alleluia! Following the amputation, I leaned back into normal life: I learned to walk on an artificial leg (prosthesis). I learned how to get dressed with a prosthesis on. I was even learning how to drive with one leg. In April, I was looking forward to my sixteenth birthday, to getting my driver's license, and to doing other sixteen-year-old things.

Every two months or so, I would get a checkup at the Mayo Clinic: blood work, X-rays, a CT scan, and a physical exam. The first two checkups confirmed that everything looked fine. In April 1981, my mom drove me to the Mayo Clinic for another checkup. This time there was bad news. There were multiple cancer nodules in both lungs—meaning that the prior November, the cancer had spread before the amputation. The drive home was pretty silent.

When we got home, Mom called Dad at work. Mom: "Del, come home." Dad: "Why?" Mom: "Just come home." My dad came home. I don't really like to recall the conversation that I had with Dad that day. I'm actually not sure that you could call it a conversation. There was a great deal of sobbing, as much of it Dad sobbing as me sobbing. Dad saying the most heartfelt and heavy things he ever said to me. Very private and personal things that I won't divulge (even after forty-three years). I still tear up just thinking about it.

The initial proclamation by Dr. Sim had been that I would live a normal life. The discovery of the cancer in my lungs gave the lie to that proclamation. The survival prognosis went down to 5 percent. Why does bone cancer that began in the legs spread to the lung? Because the cancer cells break off from the primary tumor and travel through the bloodstream until they get trapped in the very thin membranes of a lung. Once trapped, they begin to grow. If they are left untreated, they will eventually prove fatal.

30

The treatment for sarcoma nodules in the lungs is surgery—technically, a thoracotomy. In the words of one doctor, a surgeon "cracks open your chest" (literally "crack," because one's ribs often break when they are spread apart so that they can access one's lungs). The surgeon then snips out as many of the nodules as the surgical team can find. In my case, I remember that the first surgery resulted in fifteen to twenty such nodules being removed. Then they sew you back up. In order to make sure you don't develop pneumonia, physical therapists come in and pound on your chest. The entire procedure is incredibly painful.

The surgeries were so painful that after my first two thoracotomies, I told my dad, "Never again."

I was wrong.

I had many more thoracotomies. When a CT identified a nodule, they would crack open my chest and snip it out. One time, they spotted only one nodule on a scan. The surgeon went in, but couldn't find it—perhaps because of all the scar tissue. So they had to sew me up, let the nodule grow, then go back in a couple of months later. My main lung surgeon, Dr. Kaufman, felt really bad about that incident. He said two things to my mom: "I've seen them stop coming" ("them" being the cancerous metastases in my lungs). And, "I would never do anything to Rolf that I wouldn't do to my own son." That latter comment prompted my mom to cry pretty heavily. By the end of my war with cancer, I'd had at least twelve thoracotomies. I literally lost count. It's not like Mayo Clinic gives you a punch card so that every twentieth surgery is free. It's kind of fun to wonder what I would choose if I won a free surgery, though.

After the first two thoracotomies, I began chemotherapy. Even though it was forty years earlier than Mike, I received some of the same drugs that he did: Cytoxan, Adriamycin, vincristine, as well as one other, methotrexate. The Adriamycin, which can damage your heart if your lifetime dosage is high, was the worst for me—for years, I would vomit if anything smelled or even looked like it. My chemo routine went like this: After checking into the hospital, my mom would bring me a last blast of calories from the diner across the street—a chocolate-banana milkshake and a bacon, lettuce, and peanut-butter sandwich. Don't knock it until you try it as a pick-me-up in anticipation of two days of throw-up time.

This second battle in my war with cancer was when things really started to get bad. My hair fell out, my chances of survival dropped to "lower than a snake's belly" (that's a technical, medical term), and the chemotherapy was punishing. Normal life disappeared.

---

## KARL (2022)

During my first thirty-day stay in the hospital I learned two kind of surprising things. First, I learned that when you're in the hospital you never *really* rest. Oh, you may be in bed a lot, and you may sleep a lot, and you may even have a single room, but you almost never get a full night's sleep—whether this is because of discomfort, or because of treatment, or because you never sleep well if you're not in your own bed. Or because a nurse is coming in to take your vitals, or administer medicine, or ask, "Are you sleeping?" (Yes, that really happened.

32

More than once. Super helpful.) Or because the poor man in the room next door to you is battling not only cancer but dementia and thinks that the fire alarm is a camera, that he's being watched, and keeps calling for help. (Yes, that happened too.) A stay in the hospital is not restful; there's just too much going on. I didn't truly start to rest and recover until I was home again.

Second, I learned that, for all of the hustle and bustle, the hospital can be incredibly quiet. In between the hustles and amid the bustle there are eerie silences, silences that can begin to feel heavy—literal silence that can begin to press in on the emotional and spiritual silences that we might be wrestling with.

I experienced several deep silences while I was in my first stay. In those early days there was so much uncertainty. In one of my earliest conversations with my oncologist, he told me that as recently as fifteen years ago, this leukemia was a death sentence. Even now, as far as treatments have come, the survival rates are not stellar, and the recurrence rates are high. The hill ahead looked steep, the road long, the night dark, the metaphors mixed. The first silence I struggled with was relational silence. There were folks from whom I might have expected to hear something, anything, but who were silent. It was a difficult time, lonely in part because of COVID restrictions (I was allowed only one visitor a day at the beginning of it all), and in part because so many folks just don't know what to say, and so nothing gets said. This was, as it turned out, the least troubling silence for me, because it wasn't absolute, and it wasn't lasting. One of my oldest friends called me almost eighteen months after my initial diagnosis. When I picked up the phone the first thing he said was, "I'm a terrible friend; I should have called sooner." My response to him was, "Nonsense, you're calling now!" It's never too late.

The second silence that pressed in on me was my sense of God's silence. When I prayed, when I called out to God, it felt as though God wasn't answering, at least not in any way that I could *hear*. In this feeling, I knew that I wasn't alone. I turned to the Psalms, where the pray-er often complains that God is being silent. I found them helpful. Many of the prayers in the Psalms are cries for help, which beg the Lord God to break the silence. Psalm 109 begins with a plea: "Do not be silent, O God of my praise." Yet it ends with the confidence that, while the psalmist's enemies may speak curses, "you," O Lord, "will bless" (Ps. 109:1, 28). Psalm 35 calls on the Lord to bring a case against the psalmist's enemies, and to testify:

> You have seen, O LORD; do not be silent!
> O Lord, do not be far from me!
> Wake up! Bestir yourself for my defense,
> for my cause, my God and my Lord!
> (Ps. 35:22–23)

And it isn't only the psalms that do this. Jesus, in his prayer in the garden and in his cry from the cross, spoke to God's silence and begged for an answer. For me, these witnesses were tremendously comforting. What the cross and the prayers for help teach us is that silence is where God shows up most powerfully. The cross and the prayers for help, therefore, commend to us an almost paradoxical hope—that we can learn to hear God in the silence.

The third silence, which came last, was my own silence, in response to God's silence when I prayed. One of the challenges

I faced in the hospital was difficulty sleeping through the night. There was a stretch of several weeks where I would wake up, every night, at 2:00 or 2:30, and lie awake, my mind "working," or at least going. I dealt with this wakefulness during the "dark watches" of the night (Ps. 63:6), most often by praying. For a little while I fell out of the habit—the ability, the capacity—to pray. *I* fell silent.

Then one night, as I tried to pray, I learned something that ought, I suppose, to have been obvious all along. As I began to pray, I found my mind wandering, unable to focus; my "prayer" about my situation—regular chemotherapy treatments, new medications, and so on—was disjointed and incoherent. So, *I stopped, and decided to pray not for myself but for others. And wouldn't you know it, my mind settled and my focus was clear.* I prayed for my wife Angela, and for our five children; for the rest of my family; for my colleagues and the people of the congregation I was serving; for my sister's friend Joyce as she, too, faced cancer (in her case, cancer on top of cancer); for my side-by-side partner Mike, who was in the midst of what he called his own "strike days." And, prayers said, I drifted off, at peace. Now, I am not suggesting that we shouldn't pray about and for ourselves. I believe that we should. But at times praying for others is just what we need—just what I needed—to get out of our own head, out of our own way, and trust that others are praying for us too. We are part of a fraternity of prayer, and when we join in, there peace abounds.

What I learned is similar to what the pray-er of Psalm 32 says,

> While I kept silence, my body wasted away
> through my groaning all day long.

> For day and night your hand was heavy upon me;
> my strength was dried up as by the heat of
> summer. (Ps. 32:3–4)

My *body* wasn't wasting away because of my silence, but my spirit and my mood, my attitude were. When I broke my silence, my well-being was well served.

---

### MIKE (2022)

A little more than a month into treatment, I had the opportunity to go up to "the cabin" for a change of scenery. ("The cabin" is my in-laws' home, just a couple of hours north of us, and the place that has been our family's gathering place for rest, recreation, and holidays.) At least, that was the reason—a "change of scenery"—I was choosing for our outing. The real issue or concern was my immunocompromised status, a result of my initial chemo treatments. Any potential cause for a fever, even as relatively low as 100.4 degrees Fahrenheit, would earn me an automatic trip to the ER. Prior to cancer, 100.4 would've meant merely taking two Tylenol and going to bed early. Now, however, it meant a trip to the ER—which had already happened twice since my diagnosis. And with COVID still lurking, the concern was more than just the possibility for a case of the sniffles. Previously simple realities, such as a mild fever, now were a potential major reason for concern from the standpoint of a possible infection that could make me sick enough not to be able to drive. I was not supposed to be alone. So my beloved wife Kari would fuss about me being alone, much to the annoyance of my stubborn and belligerent self. After all, I'm a big boy and like to think I can take care of myself.

So the "change of scenery" at the cabin was really all about me not being alone. Kari needed to be at an overnight retreat at our Bible camp for its board of directors, on which she served. Our youngest daughter, Eleanor, who was still at home throughout this ordeal, was going to be occupied all weekend helping with tech for the middle school musical, leaving the potential for *a lot* of alone, "unsupervised" time and space for me. I was perfectly fine with that. Kari and Eleanor were not, and for good reason.

The previous Wednesday evening, Kari and Eleanor had left me alone after I assured them I would be fine for a couple of hours. It was Lent, and Kari was at her parish an hour north for worship. Eleanor was at school running tech for the middle school musical.

Unfortunately, that evening I began to feel sharp waves of pain in my lower abdomen remarkably not unlike, though not nearly as severe as, the abdominal pain that had already twice sent me to the ER leading up to my diagnosis. (I had been to the ER more over the last month than I had over the previous 53 years of my life combined.) Around suppertime I began to feel feverish. So a "fever watch" began: 99.2 ... 99.6 ... 98.7 (Whew!) ... 99.1 (Dang it!) ... 99.4 ... 100.00 (Uh oh!) ... 97.7 (That's more like it.) ... 99.3 (Here we go again.) ... and so on. My oncologist's instructions were not to take anything to reduce the fever, lest that mask an infection I might be battling. All the while, the stomach pains left me calling out and exhausted following each wave.

Fortunately, one of the sacramental blessings in my life was and continues to be my closest friends, a couple of whom have

37

been my cycling buddies who live in St. Cloud, a short half hour away. A call to Matt summoned his services: "Matt, I know how this will go: If you come and hang with me to be on standby in case I have to go to the ER, it'll be a wasted evening for you—other than getting to hang out with me in my anguish and anxiety—and nothing else will happen. But if I continue to try to tough this out, my fever will certainly hit the magic number, and I'll be in too much pain to drive myself to the ER." And of course, Matt came right away to hang out with me until Eleanor and Kari got home. And, as predicted after enough experience predicting and counter-ing Murphy's Law, with Matt's presence and Kari's eventual return and vigilance, no trip to the ER was needed. That time.

So with the potential for lots of alone time again loom-ing for the weekend, and with the most recent fever and ER escapades in mind, Kari and I headed north for a weekend of changed scenery and not-so-alone time at her folks' place. That Friday afternoon I developed an ache in my lower back, right in the middle, above my tailbone. But what started as a minor ache and a dismissive explanation (I *had* walked and carried more up and down stairs to get ready to go that morn-ing than I had in a month, I rationalized) became, after going to bed, a throb at the site and source of pain in my back, trav-eling up my spine and into my head. Eventually, after several hours of pain, finding no comfortable position in which to sleep, I broke down and took the pain pill I had been trying to avoid because of its main side effect of constipation, and I found at least a handful of hours of uninterrupted sleep. But not before the mind games started in the quiet and solitude of the night, when the voices and fears that we all carry in our hearts and heads about whatever it is we happen to be facing in life find their opportunity and volume: "Maybe this is the cancer? Maybe it's spread to my bones? (Does lymphoma even spread to bones?) What was it the oncologist had said about my 'double hit' lymphoma and recurrence in the brain . . . 5 to 7 percent? Maybe the cancer is already in my spinal fluid?" And on. And on. And on. And on.

The next day I mentioned the night's ordeal to my father-in-law, he himself a twenty-plus-year survivor of colon cancer: "In addition to last night's pain," I said, "I couldn't get my brain to turn off and let go of all the 'what-ifs'!"

"That never really goes away," he assured me.

For the most part, since my treatments had started, I had—or so I had thought—avoided many of these long, dark nights of the soul, with the exception of a full-on hyperventilating panic attack in the cab of my pickup truck, trailside, after a particularly cold fat-bike ride (one of my last) early on in the diagnosis ordeal. But whatever the label of the experience of those nights—the product of an overactive imagination? worry? fear? rationalization? preparation for the worst? all of the above?—I had also begun to discover an intentionality in calling on tools and continually growing coping mechanisms that a decade plus of crisis ministry in the parish had "provided." My faith was a bedrock foundation. And along with that faith had come faith practices established on that foundation. My faith, through decades of life and its trials, had become not just a faith in some abstract "presence" of God but a trust and hope in explicit promises in the cross of Christ, signed on my brow in the waters of baptism. I had come to believe that although death is inevitable, it will not be the final word in my life. This is true of death itself, but also of the metaphorical deaths that we experience throughout life—professional deaths, vocational deaths, relational deaths, and so on. Because of Christ, I am promised, none of these will have the last word. My faith trusts that God shows up in the here and now.

Prayer was one of the places and moments that God showed up. Prayer, especially for others—for my pal Karl, for the half dozen or so other people right around my age who were battling cancer, and more—helped me, even at times just momentarily, take my mind off myself. Deep-breathing exercises and terms and practices like "radical acceptance" that I've picked up and filed away after a bout with depression calmed my heart rate and anxiety. And, of course (shocker!), our forebears in the faith and their collection of words, experiences, and encounters with God, and prayers, all bear witness that God shows up in our prayers.

I found an encounter of God's assuring presence—that is, God showed up—in the cancer veterans in my life and their wealth of experience, who have been able to say, "Yeah, I remember that"—my father-in-law, my sister, some of my closest friends, parishioners present and past. There was an authenticity and credibility in those conversations far greater than the well-meaning knuckleheads looking for something meaningful to say who regaled me with stories of the horrible and painful death of their cousin Eddie when he got cancer. (Don't do that. Please. Far better to simply show up and "be.")

God continued to show up in the presence of my friends and our shared sense of humor that for those on the outside looking in might even tend toward the "inappropriate" or gallows end of things, recalling God's last laugh in the seemingly-delayed-yet-nonetheless-fulfilled promises to

Sarah and Abraham in the birth of their son Isaac, whose name means "laughter."

God continued to show up in the knowledge, expertise, and skill of my doctors; in the compassion and doggedness of my care coordinator, especially in handling the absurdity of far-away insurance companies and the endless questions and reminders of what doctors had ordered; in the presence and attention of all the nurses and caregivers in the cancer ward; and yes, even in the medicine pumped into my body.

Each of these and more—the presence of my wife Kari and our kids, the gift of having a place to go to rest and be renewed at the lake, the gift of technology that kept me connected with friends and family—have provided moments of not just the proverbial counted blessings life may or may not bring. More deeply, more profoundly, and more to the point of faith and its trust in God's promised presence, each of these provided point and counterpoint to the fear, worry, imagination, and rationalization that came with every perceived new lump, pain, symptom, and side effect. I was not left bereft nor abandoned in this ordeal.

———

One of the beautiful things about human beings is that we are, by nature, curious. We want to know things, to understand how things work, to learn. As with all gifts, there can be a shadow side to our curiosity; it isn't just that we want to know, but at times that we *need* to know, we *have* to understand. This can lead to some wild reactions to hard and surprising news.

*People want things to make sense.* We live in a world in which most (but not all) of our reality is a result of cause and effect. Study for the math test, and you will probably do better than if you didn't study. Play tennis against the garage, and you will eventually knock out all of the garage door window panels (we know this one by experience—sorry, Dad). Practice the piano, and you will get better at playing piano (we know this one by experience too—Mike, because he practiced; Karl and Rolf, not so much). So many things in our life are governed by cause and effect. But not all things.

Not all diseases or tragedies make sense, and they don't all happen for a reason. When we learn about a hard diagnosis or difficult news, whether we are getting it for ourselves or hearing about someone else, we often look for reasons, causes, and explanations for why something is happening. At these times, the human desire (need?) for things to make sense can be helpful. As a rule, when you hear some bad news or experience it yourself, it is best if you make an intentional effort to suspend the need for things always to make sense. Do your best to avoid searching for a cause.

When Rolf's cancer was first diagnosed, a woman from the congregation where the family belonged, where Rolf and Karl's dad served as pastor, approached Rolf's mother, Katherine, one Sunday morning. She said, "Don't you feel guilty that Rolf has cancer?" Katherine responded, "I certainly feel bad, but why would I feel guilty?" The woman then went on, "If you had served your family a diet full of fresh fruits and vegetables, Rolf wouldn't have cancer." Katherine was a short woman, all of five-foot-three at her tallest, but she slugged the woman right on the chin. Talk about punching up!

Okay, that's not true—it's just Rolf and Karl's fantasy. Katherine was incredibly kind and would never have slugged anyone. But, you know, Rolf and Karl are romantics . . . so they can wish their mom would have popped that judgy lady right on the kisser. Instead, with a certain amount of energy in her voice, Katherine simply said, "You can't pin that one on me." She never divulged the name of the woman who said this—because maybe her kids can be a little judgy too.[1]

This unnamed Christian woman wasn't being nasty, or mean-spirited, or even intentionally judgmental (well, maybe a little). Yet, in her desire to make sense of why this was happening, she leapt to a conclusion that she could wrap her mind around. She wanted to believe that a perfect diet would protect against cancer and other illnesses.[2] As if all bad things happen for a reason. Similarly, many years later, one of the best pastors we've ever known inquired about Rolf's cancer and then asked, "Did you grow up near power lines?" Even a great pastor—who should know better—wanted *a reason. A reason why bad things happen to nice people, why kids get cancer, why seemingly healthy fathers drop dead.* But life does not always make sense. Sometimes there is no cause and effect. But even so, people want there to be a reason for things.

People do this—*we* do this—all the time. Even to ourselves. A dear friend's mother developed Lou Gehrig's disease when he was a first-year seminary student. She told our friend, "I don't know what I did to cause God to give me this disease. The only thing I can think of is that I loved my kids more than I loved God." Ouch.

We even do this to ourselves. When Karl was in the ER, awaiting his diagnosis, he was wondering if he had done something to himself—drank too much, didn't exercise enough, or something—and in a strange way, felt some relief (relief!) when he learned that he had leukemia. Sometimes the desire to know the reason, to identify a cause or even a purpose, can lead to some very unhelpful lines of thinking. And unhelpful lines of speaking.

_____

KARL (2001)

As we said in the introduction, this book isn't about cancer. It starts there, for the three of us, but that's not all it is about. All of us have faced challenges and struggle and even suffering in other ways. No doubt this is a part of life. In 2001, my then-wife and I were expecting our third child. And, potentially, maybe a third and a fourth. My wife was as big as a house, and we were wondering, hoping even, that we might be expecting twins (as Minnesotans, this was doubly exciting). The ultrasound at six months told a different story. The child was already dead in utero. It was a painful drive home from the doctor's office. When we got home I called my dad to share the news. After barely getting it out, and shedding tears, I listened as my father quietly wept with me, and then he simply said, "God is in it."

Dad didn't mean, "This is God's plan," or "God has a reason," but instead that I could expect that this God of ours—who came to Mary and Martha's side when Lazarus had died, who healed a hemorrhaging woman, who raised a little girl from death, and who went to the cross and the grave for us—this God shows up when the walls of the valley of the shadow of death are closing in.

_____

When a cancer diagnosis comes, or when terrible, heartbreaking news arrives, when the night is at its darkest, look for

God to show up—*expect God to show up*. What we are getting at is the core message of the gospel—what many theologians call "the theology of the cross." The heart of the theology of the cross—or, as St. Paul calls it in 1 Corinthians 1:18, "the word of the cross" (RSV)—is a counterintuitive promise: *that the very place where God seems to be most absent—the death of the Son of God on a cross—is actually the one place in all of creation where God is most present and active!* The theology of the cross promises us that Christ Jesus comes to us, reveals himself to us, and loves us most clearly and most fully on the cross. And this was not just a one-and-done revelation. According to Paul, this is who God is and how God will continue to come to us. This is who Jesus is! As Paul writes in Philippians, quoting an early Christian hymn (and most likely adding a couple of lines to it in order to emphasize this point),

> Christ Jesus, who was in the form of God,
>> did not regard equality with God
>> as something to be exploited,
> but he emptied himself,
>> taking on the form of a slave,
>> being born in human likeness.
> And being found in human form,
>> he humbled himself
>> and became obedient to the point of death—
>> *even death on a cross!* (Phil. 2:6–8 NRSV
>> modified)

This is perhaps New Testament theology at its purest. And it is good news. It is good news for one who is facing suffering of his or her own. And, as we have all learned, this is not just theology, nor merely a doctrine; this is lived faith. It is faith at work, faith working in us, precisely in our most difficult times.

Martin Luther describes how we should look for God to show up. When the world sees Jesus on the cross, crucified, "it looks at him only as a man in his weakness"—in other words, they see the cross as the absence of God, because the world expects God to show up only in mountaintop moments. But Luther sees Paul pointing to the crucified Jesus in order "to teach us what is the true Christian religion. *It does not begin at the top, as all other religions do; it begins at the bottom.*" In order to understand how God saves and shows up, "you must put away all speculations about the Majesty, all thoughts of works, traditions, and philosophy—indeed, of the Law of God itself. And you must run directly to the manger and the mother's womb, embrace this Infant and Virgin's Child in your arms, and look at Him—born, being nursed, growing up, going about in human society, teaching, dying, rising again."[3]

A vulnerable child born to a virgin in a cattle stall and placed in the animals' feeding trough. An innocent man nailed to a cross and left to die. That's where God has chosen to show up. Which means that we should learn to look for God to show up not only in life's highest highs but also in life's lowest lows. Especially in life's lows!

The three of us are pastors. We have been called to many hospital rooms, to many deathbeds, to many funeral homes, and to many gravesides. And the three of us have experienced a recurring phenomenon that we now have come to expect. It goes like this:

- "I entered the hospital room expecting to minister to them, but they ministered to me."
- "I went to the deathbed to offer hope, but they were already filled with hope."
- "I went to the funeral home to speak of new life, but life was already there."
- "I went to the graveside to preach to them, but I found that they were preaching to me."

And so on. All of these examples—and every other pastor that we know well has described similar experiences—point to the reality that God shows up in our suffering. This is where the rubber meets the road, and where God—in Christ Jesus—comes to us most powerfully as Immanuel, "God with us."

The reality that God is with us powerfully in the midst of our own suffering means that a very different form of prayer is given to us—a form of prayer in which we can complain vigorously, lament powerfully, and shout-pray for God to show up: "God with us!" What, then, does this mean for us as we face mortality, suffering, and the threat of death? Just this: If we can expect God to show up, and yet are struggling with what feels like God's silence, or absence, then we can *demand* that God show up.

This is, of course, the complete opposite of "When God closes one door, God opens another." The fundamental nature of doors is that, if they are closed, they can be opened again. If you feel like God is closing a door for you, don't go looking for a different door, or a window to climb through. Ball up your fist and *knock on the door*. Hammer on it. Scream at God. Say, "Open this door!" Say, "This is how doors work, O God. They close and then they open. They close again and open again! Open! This! Door!"

In the book of Psalms, the demand that God answer is often made. Several times the plea is that God do so quickly, speedily, *now*! Psalm 69 offers one of the fullest expressions of this demand:[4]

> As for me, my prayer is to you, O LORD.
> At an acceptable time, O God,
>     in the abundance of your steadfast love,
>         answer me.
> With your faithful help rescue me
>     from sinking in the mire;
> let me be delivered from my enemies
>     and from the deep waters.
> Do not let the flood sweep over me,
>     or the deep swallow me up,
>     or the Pit close its mouth over me.
> Answer me, O LORD, for your steadfast love is good;
>     according to your abundant mercy, turn to me.
> Do not hide your face from your servant,
>     for I am in distress—make haste to answer me.
> Draw near to me, redeem me,
>     set me free because of my enemies. (Ps. 69:13–18)

Notice that in calling on God to answer, the pray-er of this psalm first says, "at an acceptable time," and then adds, "make haste." The acceptable time for God may be later, but for the one praying, that time is now. Part of the pain of living with illness is living with the distance between our "acceptable time" and God's "acceptable time." Or maybe it is about living

48

*within* the distance between our acceptable time and God's. Perhaps the question is as simple as this: What does it mean to say to God, "Make haste to answer me," and then live in the long silence when it seems God is not making haste?

One of the most important things that we learned about prayer in our journeys and in our studies is that we need to let go of the idea that prayer is only a wish list of "asks" that we bring before God and that we expect God to "answer." Prayer is more than asking for things—prayer *is* about bringing our pleas before God, but it is about more than that. Prayer consists of our words spoken in response to God, who has first spoken to us. Eugene Peterson offers one of the most important words of wisdom about prayer that we have learned: "Prayer is never the first word; it is always the second word. God has the first word. Prayer is answering speech; it is not primarily 'address' but 'response.' Essential to the practice of prayer is fully to realize this secondary quality."[5] Peterson adds, "Prayer is the human word and is never the first word, never the primary word, never the initiating and shaping word simply because we are never first, never primary. We do not honor prayer by treating it as something that it is not, even when that something is, as we suppose, sacred and exalted."[6]

Through our wars with cancer, through our years of ministry, through our experiences of praying for ourselves and others, Peterson's wise insight has been confirmed. When we conceive of prayer primarily as a wish list or a set of asks, we reduce prayer to our own activity, our own speech. Prayer is a secondary word—our word in response to the One who spoke the beloved creation into existence: "God said, 'Let there be light'; and there was light. And God saw that the light was good" (Gen. 1:3–4a). Prayer is response to Jesus, who *is* the Word of God. God not only spoke creation into existence, God the Speaker spoke a Word of life, love, and liberation to creation. The name of that Word is Jesus—the same Jesus who died on a cross in order that we might have life.

When we understand prayer as "secondary speech," we then conceive of prayer not as just a wish list but as a way of connecting our lives to the life of the One who suffered, who died, and who was raised from death in order that we might have abundant life. Prayer is a way of inviting the One who suffered into our suffering. Especially when we pray out of the midst of our own suffering and the suffering of others, prayer is a way—*the* way!—of drawing God into our lives and ourselves into God's life. We will let Peterson have the last word on prayer for now:

> We want life on our conditions, not on God's conditions. Praying puts us at risk of getting involved in God's conditions. . . . Praying most often doesn't get us what we want but what God wants, something quite at variance with what we conceive to be in our best interests. And when we realize what is going on, it is often too late to go back.[7]

# 3

# Meals and Milestones

## How We Show Up for Each Other

You prepare a table before me
   in the presence of my enemies;
you anoint my head with oil;
   my cup overflows.

             —Psalm 23:5

I am cringe-worthy to my adversaries,
   Even more so to my neighbors,
A horror to those who know me,
   Those who see me on the street turn from me.

             —Psalm 31:11 (our translation)

---

**ROLF (1981)**

The worst part of the worst part of my life was the six months between October 1981 and March 1982—my junior year in high school. I was sixteen.

They had already amputated my right leg. But the cancer had spread to my lungs. I had already endured four lung surgeries and a summer of chemotherapy. Then came the truly devastating news.

My left leg had also developed cancer. A second primary occurrence of the bone cancer. What are the odds?

When I reported to the doctors at Mayo Clinic that I suspected my left leg had also developed cancer, they reassured me, "It's natural that you might fear that, but it isn't possible. It's never happened before." Long story short, doctors no longer can say, "It's never happened before." It happened to me. And since, it has happened to a dozen or more others. What *are* the odds?

The doctors tried to save my leg. Big mistake. But they didn't know any better. After all, it had never happened before. An initial bone scan detected no sign of cancer in my leg. But it was there. It continued to grow. By the time I went back in and said I was sure there was cancer in my leg, the tumor had grown very large. In October, the doctors prescribed a course of radiation, which they hoped would reduce the tumor enough so that they could cut it out and insert a titanium knee.

During the course of radiation, I stayed in the Northland House (later a Ronald McDonald House)—a home in which kids fighting cancer could stay along with their parents. I would have daily radiation, and my dad or mom would stay with me.

On one occasion, my dad was staying with me. He announced, "Jerry Larson is coming down today, and he is going to take us out to dinner."

I replied, "No. I don't feel well enough to go to dinner. You go out with Jerry. I'll just stay here and have a bath." Dad said okay.

But Dad's friend Jerry was a powerful force of nature. And like many a force of nature, Jerry was an irresistible force. Jerry was a traveling salesman who sold paper (legal pads, typing paper, notebook paper) and related products to college bookstores. His clients loved him because he loved life. He wore a smile and exuded enthusiasm for almost everything in life. He probably stood a hair shy of six feet tall. And when I say "a hair shy," I mean that quite literally. Jerry had male-pattern baldness—a clean horseshoe of aging blond hair crowned his bald dome. He tried to bargain with his barber that he should only have to pay half price for a haircut. His complexion always seemed to run bright red. Jerry carried a bit of extra weight around his middle. His reddish skin tone may have been the result of his elevated blood pressure, his joy for life, or both.

Jerry insisted that I join him and Dad for dinner. And when Jerry insisted, well, I was no match. They loaded me into the back seat of his traveling-salesman sedan. The tumor had swelled to the point at which I could not fully bend my knee, so I had to sit sideways in the back seat, with my leg up on the bench seat. My leg was dully throbbing with low-level pain. But my brain. My brain was raging. I did not want to go out to dinner. So as Jerry drove, I was sideways. I was sitting sideways. And my mood was even more sideways. I would endure dinner, and later, I would let Dad know how much I hated it.

Jerry guided the sedan north of Rochester to a county supper club called the Fisherman's Inn. We were seated, and the waitress came over. Dad and Jerry ordered a beer, and I ordered a Pepsi. She returned with our drinks and asked if we had any questions about the menu. It was a Minnesota supper club, so they probably had a special with a baked potato. I can't recall exactly. But what happened next I remember quite vividly.

Jerry asked, "How are your ribs?"

She replied flatly, "They're good."

Jerry repeated, "No, I mean, *how are your ribs*?"

She answered with a little more emphasis, "Our ribs are good."

Jerry fired back, "You're not getting my question, I want to know if your ribs are really good."

She tried a third time, "Our ribs are really good."

Jerry piled on, "If your favorite uncle were coming to town . . . I mean your favorite uncle! When you were a little girl he would do anything for you and now that you are grown up, you would do anything for him. You've got other uncles, but he is your favorite. And now he's in town, and he's coming to dinner here. And his favorite food in the world is ribs. *Would you let him eat the ribs here?*"

The waitress caught the spirit of the show Jerry was putting on. I don't know if she just decided to play along or if she actually believed what she said next. But looking him in the eye, she exclaimed, "I would *insist* that he have our ribs!"

"We're all having ribs!" Jerry cried out. And we did. The ribs were great—just the right balance of protein, carbs, and fat that an emaciated cancer kid needed. The meal as a whole was even better. There probably was a baked potato; I can't remember. But Jerry's enthusiasm, laughter, joy for life, and love were transformative. The whole experience of that meal— the food, the friendship, the fun—turned me inside out. Prior to the meal, I was quietly enraged that I had been dragged along. After the meal, I was *thankful* for Jerry's irresistible invitation. Prior to the meal, I was understandably focused on the slow throb of the tumor (it really was unpleasant). After the meal, I was *grateful* for the magnificent intrusion into the day-after-day grind of radiation. Prior to the meal, I was living a life of isolation and scarcity. I was at Mayo Clinic—away from family, away from friends, away from home. The only thing I was looking forward to each day was a hot bath. The meal was a brief but wonderful experience of abundance and community in the midst of the scarcity and isolation.

I look back on that meal as the best moment in the worst part of my life. It is not an overstatement to say that I am (almost) eternally grateful to Jerry and to God for that moment.

In November, they cut out the cancer by cutting the bone above and below the knee and inserting a metal knee. The hope was that the flesh would heal around the replacement knee. Unfortunately, the radiation had badly damaged the tissue in my leg and the wound would not heal. From November through April I was confined to bed, while they continued to give me chemotherapy and lung surgeries to fish the cancer out of my lungs. During this time, the leg never healed well enough for me to stand and eventually recurring infections became a problem.

The caregivers at Mayo Clinic tried to save my leg for almost six months. But all the king's horses and all the king's men . . . On March 13, 1982, they amputated my second leg. The battle to save my legs was over. I lost. It was time to get into a wheelchair and get on with life.

———

According to the Gospel of John, Jesus came that we might have life—abundant life. Jesus said, "I came that they may

have life, and have it abundantly" (John 10:10b). Jesus is
about far more than living right. Jesus is even about more
than salvation. Jesus is about abundant life.

But in the midst of suffering, experiencing abundant life
can be difficult. When you're too sick to stand up. When
the chemotherapy is making you vomit and lose your hair.
When death is near or overwhelming grief and sadness take
your appetite away. In these and many other similar cases,
experiencing abundant life can seem impossible. So one has
to work at creating experiences of abundant life—as my dad's
friend Jerry did when he took us out for ribs.

When the Bible wants to give a picture of God's abundance
or of the abundant life, one of the most common metaphors it
employs is the feast. In Isaiah 25, the prophet sees a vision of
the future in which God's reign is so completely achieved that
even death itself is defeated ("swallowed up," v. 8). Seeking to
capture the abundance of that promised future, the prophet
paints a picture of a grand feast. Here is Eugene Peterson's
translation of Isaiah 25:6–8 (The Message):

> But here on this mountain,
>     God-of-the-Angel-Armies
>     will throw a feast for all the people of the world,
> A feast of the finest foods, a feast with vintage wines,
>     a feast of seven courses, a feast lavish with
>         gourmet desserts.
> And here on this mountain, God will banish
>     the pall of doom hanging over all peoples,
> The shadow of doom darkening all nations.
>     Yes, he'll banish death forever.
> And God will wipe the tears from every face.
>     He'll remove every sign of disgrace

From his people, wherever they are.
　　Yes! GOD says so!

According to the prophet Isaiah, when God's promised-and-preferred future of abundant life breaks in, it will be a feast. A feast with the best food—the finest meats and cheeses; the best beer, wine, and soda; desserts of chocolate, fruit, and cream. A feast with the entire world invited. A feast of joy and abundance.

According to the Scriptures, God desires that from time to time (not all of the time) we should experience the joy of divine abundance in the form of a feast. The Old Testament includes this law:

> Every year, set aside 10 percent of the entire harvest of your crops that is brought in from the field. In the presence of the LORD your God, in the place that he will choose as a dwelling for his name [Jerusalem], you shall eat the 10 percent of your grain, your wine, and your olive oil, as well as the firstborn of your herd and flock, *so that you may learn to revere the LORD your God always.*
>
> [Or, if you live a long way from Jerusalem], you may exchange the 10 percent for money. With the money securely in your hand, go to the place that the LORD your God will choose [Jerusalem]. *Spend the money for whatever you wish—oxen, sheep, wine, beer, or whatever you desire.* And you shall eat there in the presence of the LORD your God, you and your household rejoicing together. As for the Levitical priests who live in your towns, do not neglect them, because they have no land or inheritance with you. (Deut. 14:22–27; our translation)

When this passage was read in chapel at the seminary that all three of us attended, an older, pious professor loudly exclaimed, "*That's in the Bible?!*" You bet it is! Once in a while (here, once a year), God desires that we feast on the goodness of creation. Why? So that "you may learn to revere the LORD your God always" and so that "you and your household together" shall rejoice. Oh, and don't forget to invite the pastors and others who don't have as much as you do: "the homeless, the orphans, and the widows" in your neighborhood (v. 29; our translation). If we don't feast once in a while on the abundance of God's creation, we won't learn to revere and worship the Lord in a proper, biblical way. The great Christian leader Tony Campolo explains the biblical logic as follows:

> It is in partying that we know a little something about the kind of God we have. He is not some kind of transcendental Shylock demanding His pound of flesh; He is not some kind of deistic chairperson of the universe. Our God is a party deity. He loves a party. If you don't believe me, then just pay attention to what His Son Jesus has to say about his Father's Kingdom:
>
>> The kingdom of heaven is like unto a certain king, which made a marriage for his son, And sent forth his servants to call them that were bidden to the wedding: and they would not come. (Matt. 22:2–4)
>> And he saith unto me, Write, Blessed are they which are called unto the marriage supper of the Lamb. And he saith unto me, These are the true sayings of God. (Rev. 19:9)

Did you get that? Jesus says the Kingdom is like a wedding reception and He wants His friends to celebrate with Him as though He were the bridegroom.[1]

Perhaps the most beloved of all psalms is Psalm 23—the so-called Good Shepherd Psalm. The psalm's opening lines are loved: "The LORD is my shepherd, I shall not want. . . . Even though I walk through the darkest valley, I fear no evil; for you are with me." The images of God as a shepherd are loved: leading the sheep through dry and dangerous land and finding them lush, green grass to eat and sweet, cold water to drink. The images in the second half of the psalm are less familiar, but equally important.

> You prepare a table before me
>    in the presence of my enemies;
> you anoint my head with oil;
>    my cup overflows. (Ps. 23:5)

Here, the image shifts again to a meal. A meal of hospitality and honor, in which the Lord is the host of the meal. The Lord grants the place of honor at this divine feast to the one praying. And not just a place of honor next to God—but a place of honor *in the presence of one's enemies.*

The Old Testament world was a culture of honor and shame. Honor and shame were public forms of social currency. It was a person's job to gain honor for their house and their tribe. And it was a person's obligation to avoid accruing shame for their house and their tribe. Because honor and shame were social currencies, they were public. Other people in your city or country knew who was honorable and who was shameful.

The psalm paints the picture of the Lord giving you the seat of honor at the Lord's table. For the Lord to do so precisely in a setting in which your enemies would see it was an ultimate picture of honor and shame.

Students and others who don't have any personal enemies often ask how to interpret the enemies in the psalms. What if we consider the devil our enemy? What if we consider evil our enemy? What if we consider cancer, or illness, or grief, or death our enemy?

One thing to take seriously about illness and suffering is that they can create a sense of shame. I once was strong and proud of it; now I'm weak and ashamed of it. I once was healthy and proud of it; now I'm sick and embarrassed about it. I once was self-sufficient and proud of it; now I'm diminished; now I'm disabled; now I need help—it is humiliating.

At the depth of a serious illness such as cancer, there can be truly humiliating moments. Moments when you need help going to the bathroom. Moments when you have to strip naked in front of strangers, to be poked and prodded and have your least flattering features exposed. Moments when your body doesn't work. It can feel dishonorable.

Here is the thing about God. God loves honoring the dishonorable, giving a place of pride to those who have been shamed, granting glory to those who have been embarrassed.

One of the things Jerry Larson did for Rolf by putting on a show for the waitress—"How are your ribs?"—was to create a joyful moment of light in the darkest season of Rolf's life. And by picking up the check at the end of the meal, he was showering a little bit of honor on Rolf in the midst of all the shame and embarrassment Rolf was experiencing. The next day, Rolf was back in the belly of the beast, disrobing for radiation. But for a moment, through Jerry, the Lord prepared a place of honor for Rolf in the presence of his enemy—cancer. His cup overflowed.

One of the things people who are going through suffering can do is create moments of abundance, such as a great meal, a feast, or some other experience of God's wonderful creation. One of the things that caregivers can offer to their loved ones who are going through suffering is an experience of honor, of abundance, of joy, of love. The Lord sets a table for us in the midst of our suffering, in the presence of our enemies.

---

### ROLF (1991)

I was ordained as a pastor in 1991. Around the time I was ordained, a family friend who was in his late twenties suffered a sudden and massive medical event. The young man was one of four boys in a really fine family—faithful, kind, generous, cheerful. He was a teacher, had a wonderful girlfriend, and had most of life in front of him. And then the medical event. The exact nature of the event isn't important for this story. What is important is that the medical event left the young man with little brain function. Our dad, Del, is also a pastor. He met with the family, walked with them through the difficult days, and then said, "It's time to let this boy go." The medical staff removed medical support, and the boy died.

His parents went back home and did what people do in such cases—tried to go on living in the midst of inconsolable grief. They reported the following incident to us, which I will relate as accurately as I can remember it.

They were walking together in the downtown of the small, prairie town in which they lived. As they were making their way down the street, a man from their church came around the corner ahead of them—walking with his head down. As he turned the corner, he glanced up and saw them. He flinched visibly. Then turned to cross the street away from them. The man took two steps, then his shoulders slumped. And then the man did an incredible thing. He turned back to the grieving couple and approached them.

"You probably saw me when I saw you—at first I turned away from you," he admitted.

"Yes, we saw that."

"I am really sorry I did that. And I'm even more sorry about your son. I turned away at first because I don't know what to say. I still don't know what to say," he added.

"Thanks," the couple said. "Thanks for turning back to us."

One of the psalm passages that we listed at the start of this chapter goes like this:

> I am cringe-worthy to my adversaries,
>     Even more so to my neighbors,
> A horror to those who know me,
>     Those who see me on the street turn from me.
>         (Ps. 31:11; our translation)

It is almost as if this verse was written to speak for our family friends—the couple who lost their son: "Those who see me on the street turn from me." The truth is, *this psalm verse actually was written to speak for them—and to speak for anyone who has had an experience of suffering that has caused other people to cringe and turn away.*

Here is a deep truth about human nature. The human reaction of cringing and turning away from suffering is completely natural. It is a perfectly natural human emotion to feel the need to protect one's own emotional health by turning away from someone else's pain—from someone else's deep pain. Each of us has experienced this in our own lives. At times, we have been the suffering person whose pain has repelled others. As we have gone through various difficult things—cancer, divorce, miscarriage, unemployment, disability, physical disfigurement, and the like—others have at times cringed and turned away from us. And that emotional reaction is normal. Each of us has also had times when we have cringed and turned away from the suffering and pain of others. And that emotional reaction is also normal.

But here is an even deeper truth about Christian community. The Christian community experiences that emotional reaction to retreat from the suffering of others . . . and members of the Christian community do what the man on that small-town street did: They turn back and go anyway. Even if the only thing they have to say is, "I don't know what to say." Here is a hint. Go to the suffering and say, "I don't know what to say, other than that I love you. And I'm sorry."

---

In the last chapter, we said that God shows up in our suffering. You can expect that when you suffer, your God will be there—you can count on it. That is the promise of the cross.

The Christian community is called to join God by showing up for the suffering, in the midst of their suffering. So how do we join God in showing up for our family, friends, and neighbors when they are suffering? When it comes to showing up in other people's suffering, there are some dos and some don'ts.

A primary don't is this: *Do not provide easy answers—or really any answers—for why something bad is happening to a good person.*

As we discussed in the previous chapter, it is natural for us to look for answers, reasons, or explanations for much of life, especially when bad things happen. But it is vital that we never reduce someone's struggles to "answers," especially if they are simple or superficial answers— especially if they are *our* answers. Join them in their struggle. In the book of Job, the main character—Job, obviously—loses everything. Then Job's friends show up. At first, Job's friends show up and just sit with Job. "They sat with him on the ground seven days and seven nights, *and no one spoke a word to him, for they saw that his suffering was very great*" (Job 2:13). It may be that in those first days, Job's friends were at their best.

But then they opened their mouths and started talking.

The reality is that people want to say something—but sometimes they should keep quiet. When we need a reason, and cannot find one, we have a tendency to lean on the idea that God surely has a reason, one that is beyond us now but that will be revealed or can be figured out. And we tend to operate that way when people dear to us are struggling. So, you've probably heard people say things like this (and maybe said them yourself):

*Everything happens for a reason.* (Or its kissing cousin: God has a purpose [or plan] for everything.) Rolf's friend Kate Bowler, who also is a cancer survivor, wrote a famous book about her diagnosis called *Everything Happens for a Reason:*

*And Other Lies I Have Loved.*[2] She first wrote about her experience in a *New York Times* article in 2016. There Bowler describes how "a neighbor knocked on our door to tell my husband that everything happens for a reason."

> "I'd love to hear it," my husband said.
>
> "Pardon?" she said, startled.
>
> "I'd love to hear the reason my wife is dying," he said, in that sweet and sour way he has.
>
> My neighbor wasn't trying to sell him a spiritual guarantee. But there was a reason she wanted to fill that silence around why some people die young and others grow old and fussy about their lawns. She wanted some kind of order behind this chaos. Because the opposite of #blessed is leaving a husband and a toddler behind, and people can't quite let themselves say it: "Wow. That's awful." There has to be a reason, because without one we are left as helpless and possibly as unlucky as everyone else.[3]

Bowler points to the desire for "some kind of order behind the chaos" and the need to "fill that silence." Sometimes, a person should just give a hug and say, "I love you."

*When God closes a door, God opens a window.* (Or its kissing cousin: When God closes one door, God opens another.) By the way, as a person in a wheelchair, Rolf has long wondered what good it is when God opens a window after closing a door. How is the person in the wheelchair supposed to get out a window? Thanks, God, for opening the window. Sure is a lot of help!

*God will never give you more than you can handle.* We think one word responds to this saying: suicide. If God never gives people more than they can handle, why do some people die by suicide? We are heartbroken with and for anyone who has been impacted by suicide.

*Whatever doesn't kill me makes me stronger.* The German philosopher Friedrich Nietzsche wrote this. Well, actually, he wrote, "Was mich nicht umbringt, macht mich stärker."[4] He was German, after all. And he was wrong. We can definitely tell you that the chemotherapy made us all weaker. All of the surgeries (especially the amputations) made Rolf weaker. The bone marrow transplant made Karl weaker and more vulnerable. Sure, maybe we are a bit more resilient—a bit. And surely we have learned some things about how to suffer and how to find joy in the midst of sadness. But we are definitely weaker. We still cry like babies when we get a cold or COVID and sit around feeling sorry for ourselves.

*Every cloud has a silver lining.* The problem is that the opposite may be just as true: Every silver lining has a cloud. Attitude is important, but a good or healthy attitude is not a cure for illness, or a preventative; it helps, but it isn't "the answer."

And there are many others like these. Most of the time these things are said with good intentions, but you know what they say about good intentions . . .

There are (at least) two problems with this sort of thing. First, while intended to be comforting, these sorts of spiritual platitudes are often more unsettling. They can beg questions that might torment someone who is already suffering: What kind of plan is this that God has for me? or What kind of God has a plan for me like this? or Did I do something to deserve this?

Second, and more importantly, words that seek to get at a reason or understanding can, if we are not careful, come across as a push to acceptance, to get past suffering, or to "get over it." As we said in the introduction, suffering is ugly, and when we see it, we often want to turn away. Suffering repulses, and we want to get away from it and, at our best, to help others get through it.

But when people are suffering, and there is nothing substantive that we can do to make it stop, what they need is for us to be present with them in their suffering. This, once again, is a matter of faithfulness. The hard work of entering with someone into their suffering, to sit with them, wait with them, hope and cry and in fact suffer alongside them—that, too, is faithfulness.

So, what *do* we have to say?

---

## KARL (2022)

This may sound crazy, but I was a little disappointed that nobody said anything to me that was particularly pious, or foolish, or well-intentioned in a "God has a porpoise" sort of way. I say that I was disappointed because I came out of my first three months in the hospital locked and loaded and ready to go. Oh, my responses—well, comebacks . . . er, let's be honest, *rebukes*—of what I expected to be bad theology or poor spiritual care and counsel were lined up. I was ready to go off. And it never happened. Not. Once.

What I did hear from family and friends was simple, genuine, and profoundly helpful. My favorite example came from one of my dearest high school pals, Greg Moore. After high school Greg and I were in touch; we went to different colleges but saw each other from time to time. We were at each other's weddings. As will happen, over time we drifted, but one of the blessings of Facebook (yes, there are some blessings that come from Facebook and other social media) was that we reconnected and were in touch that way. When I was diagnosed in 2022, I hadn't seen Greg in person since our twenty-fifth reunion in 2013. But when Greg saw my first CaringBridge post, he was one of the first people to reach out. But not on CaringBridge. In those first days in the hospital, Greg blew up my phone with Facebook Messenger videos. Two-minute videos, five days a week (I guess he took the weekends off because being my friend is a lot like a full-time job). Even if I didn't respond, Greg sent a two-minute video Monday through Friday. Sometimes over a cup of coffee in the kitchen, sometimes over a cup of coffee on the way to work, sometimes over a cup of coffee in his garage. Cups of coffee and communication via video, what a lifeline this was, a lifeline to the real, normal, everyday world. (Greg later started introducing these videos as "Coffee with Karl," and I could tell by the way he said it that he didn't get all cute and change the *c* in "coffee" to a *k*. It's all in the pronunciation.) Greg continued to do this for eighteen months, long after both of my hospital stays, and through my recovery from transplant.

But in a really critical way, the tone of the very first video was the most memorable. Greg didn't mess around. No platitudes, no forced spirituality, just honesty. As I remember, it went something like this: "Hey, Karl, I know this is a really hard time for you. Wish I could be there. I don't have the words, I don't really know what to say. So, let me show you what I'm doing in my basement." After which he flipped the orientation of the camera around and took me on a virtual tour of his basement, which he was remodeling, putting in a work-from-home space, a bit of a "man cave," and hanging '80s movie posters (including Michael Keaton's *Batman*, or as Greg would say, Jack Nicholson's Joker). This was a simple connection, but it was in a real way one of the most important, meaningful, and life-giving pieces in those early days. It was fantastic.

In the first chapter, Mike talked about his sense of how God showed up for him in the midst of his suffering in a sacramental type of way. This "occurred through the efforts, well-wishes, cards, meals, phone calls, and visits from my family." We might call this the "Sacrament of Showing Up," where we embody, in a sense, the presence of God for our suffering loved one. Or, to put it the way Psalm 23 does, we might think of ourselves as embodying the "goodness and mercy" of God that follows, literally pursues, those whom God, and we, love.

Make no mistake, you are not a sacrament, not literally, but you can function sacramentally, bringing the grace of God with you when you show up. This may sound like a tall order, like a deadly serious responsibility. And, on the one hand, it is (although maybe we should call it a "lifely serious" responsibility). On the other hand, it can be, and perhaps should be, remarkably simple.

---

## ROLF (AROUND 2010)

I serve as a professor at Luther Seminary—a school where we educate pastors and other leaders for the Christian church, especially the Evangelical Lutheran Church in America (ELCA). One of the great—I would even say *legendary*—pastors of the ELCA in northern Minnesota was an old saint named Bob Dahlen. Bob graduated from Luther Seminary a couple of years before I started there as a student, but a few professors were already (still?) rehashing stories about Bob. Some of the brightest and best students were sent to Bob's care to serve their internship under his wise eyes. Bob served one congregation his entire ministry— a congregation in Goodridge, Minnesota, about five hours north of Minneapolis–St. Paul. Because some of the kids who were growing up in the church Bob served in Goodridge had never gone to a major metropolitan area, every couple of years Bob would bring his confirmation class down to the Twin Cities, where Bob would take them to worship at the Roman Catholic cathedral and a Jewish synagogue; to visit the Minnesota State Capitol, where they could see the battle flag of the Twenty-Eighth Virginia Infantry Regiment that the First Minnesota Infantry Regiment had captured at the battle of Gettysburg; to eat at a White Castle (because the Lutheran Reformation started at Wittenburg, aka "White-castle"); and to tour Luther Seminary. In the early days, Bob would have them spend an hour with one of our most influential teachers—Jim Nestingen, Don Juel, Gerhard Forde, or Sheldon Tostengard. Eventually, they all retired, so Bob asked me to meet with his kids when they toured.

Over the years when the kids would come, Bob and I tried several different strategies to get their attention—Bible studies, question and answer, planned discussions, presentations, and so on. I have to admit, nothing worked. I had nothing that would engage these kids—I was nowhere as interesting as the synagogue, the cathedral, the capitol, or the First Minnesota. I also have to acknowledge how phenomenally respectful these kids were—every single one of them tried very hard to be engaged. But what does a seminary professor have to say that will engage a great group of kids?

The very last time that Bob brought the kids before he retired played out pretty much the same as every other visit, until the last ten minutes. We fed the kids boxed lunches and had a discussion. After boring the kids for fifty-five minutes—one girl was hiding a bag of Cheetos under the table and sneaking bites into her mouth—I suggested that we wind the conversation down early. Bob agreed and announced that before going to White Castle, they were going to visit another man, who also happened to have no legs. Suddenly, I had an inspiration.

"Bob, before you leave, I have one more thing to say." The kids didn't look excited, but none of them visibly rolled their eyes. I said, "How many of you are fifteen years old?" A few raised their hands. "And how many of you hope to be fifteen years old someday?" The rest raised their hands. I continued.

"When I was fifteen years old, I developed cancer, and they amputated my right leg. The cancer then spread to my lungs, and eventually they also had to amputate my left leg too. All in all, I had over twenty surgeries in high school. And I want you to know something—I had the best friends in the world. I had a close group of friends that were simply wonderful, just incredible friends. During those years, how many times do you think that my closest group of friends came to see me in the hospital after a surgery?"

The girl who was sneaking Cheetos from underneath the table looked up with bright eyes, smiled, and naively exclaimed, "Every day!" There was a moment of silence and some of her classmates nodded in agreement.

"Almost never," I said. "Almost never. Do you know why?" The kids were absolutely silent. So I continued, "Because they loved me, and they didn't want to see me in pain, all hooked up to tubes and wires. Nobody who is normal wants to see someone who is in pain. Plus, they had their own lives—school, sports, band, jobs, girlfriends—and the Mayo Clinic was a ninety-minute drive from my hometown. When I was home from the hospital, they would come see me at my house all the time. They would pick me up and bring me to their homes to play games and hang out. They would encourage me and take me with them to go out. They were the best friends ever. But they almost never came to see me in the hospital, because nobody wants to be around others who are in extreme pain. I even asked my best friend, 'Why don't you come to see me in the hospital?' He responded, 'I don't like to see you that way.'"

I looked around the room, and every set of eyes in the room was pinned on me. In the last ten minutes of Bob's last visit, I'd finally found something useful to say to those fine kids.

"Understand why," I said. "If you are a normal human being, the intense, psychic pain of another person will repel you—it will push you away. It pushes me away. None of us *want* to be around those who are in pain—we don't know what to do, and we don't know what to say. So here is what I want you to do when one of your friends is in deep pain. When one of your friends has a grandparent die, or has parents get divorced, or gets cancer, or is injured in a car accident, this is what I want you to do. First, *admit to yourself* that you may not want to go. There is nothing wrong with you if you feel that. Second, *go anyway. Go anyway.*"

Then, looking at the girl with the Cheetos, I added, "And bring Cheetos. Say to your friend, 'I'm here because I love you. And I brought you some Cheetos.' Can you do that?"

They looked around the room at each other . . . and they nodded.

I'm a preacher, and I usually know a good sermon when I hear one. I even know a good sermon when it accidentally comes out of my own mouth. So, I took that simple message, and I developed it into a standard lecture and presentation that I give at Luther Seminary. "Other people's psychic pain repels us. So when a loved one is in pain, admit that you don't want to go. Then go and say, 'I love you, and I brought Cheetos.'"

I have given the talk many times in many places. And I hear back from former students and pastors, "Rolf, there was a tragedy in our congregation. And the Cheetos thing worked again."

Just before the pandemic, in 2018 or 2019, I even traveled to Princeton, Minnesota, and gave "The Cheetos Speech" at the congregation my friend Mike Pancoast was serving.

---

## MIKE (2022)

"Go. Say I love you and little else. And bring Cheetos." So said Rolf in his presentation to our confirmands at Trinity-Princeton, a teaching that continued to be repackaged into my own "good sermons," admittedly, shamelessly "ripping off" Rolf's story and points. (Isn't imitation the highest form of flattery?) But there isn't a preacher alive who doesn't at some point wonder if anything they say strikes home and sticks, if any seeds scattered seemingly willy-nilly through their preaching find any good soil at all.

My last sermon to my congregation in Princeton immediately before going on medical disability leave came on Transfiguration Sunday, February 27, 2022, and the text according to the Narrative Lectionary we followed was from John 9 and its account of Jesus's healing of the man born blind, which I paired with Matthew's account of Jesus's mountaintop transfiguration (Matt. 17).

In John's healing story, of course, sight and the ability to see are front and center. But the narrative begins with a question of causality: "Who sinned . . . ?" (John 9:2). The disciples are asking about a man born blind. According to their first-century understanding of things, suffering and calamity are brought on directly through God's immediate judgment of committed sin, either by the sufferer himself, or even the sufferer's parents or grandparents or great-grandparents. I mean, really, if we go down that road, where does one stop on the family tree—how far back does one go to discover the source of one's suffering in response to some family member's sin? We might even imagine more questions, as well: Does this generational punishment for sin carry over only between generations? Is it transmittable, say, between siblings? (If so, I'd blame my sister!)

Of course, Jesus nips that nonsense in the bud: "That's not how any of this works," he essentially says, refusing to join in the speculation around the source of the man's blindness, instead inviting consideration about what kind of response this man's blindness might elicit, and ultimately getting to work to address the man's suffering.

Throughout John's Gospel, there's "sight" and then there's "sight," and it turns out that the man born blind, ironically

enough, is the one *who truly sees Jesus*, whose darkness is en-
lightened by the Light of the World, whose faith bears witness to what he has seen—"'Yes, Lord, I believe!' . . . And he
worshiped Jesus" (9:38 NLT)—only after he has been *told*
what has happened to him, interestingly enough. Yes, he can
*see*, but it's only after Jesus *speaks* to him: "Who is he, sir? I
want to believe in him," the man who was blind inquires.
"You have seen him," Jesus said, "and he is speaking to you!"
(9:36–37 NLT). *Then* he not only sees; the man also *"sees"*
and *believes* and *worships*. The power of God's spoken Word,
the power of God's Word made flesh in Jesus, the gift of faith
that grants the eyes in our heads as well as "the eyes" of our
hearts and minds the ability to see Jesus—all of this is what
is at stake in the text from John.

This dynamic between faith and sight continues in the
events surrounding Jesus's transfiguration, where the boundaries between the visible and the invisible, between the
earthly and the heavenly, between the mundane—even the
profane—and the holy, become mysteriously, terrifyingly,
and gloriously thin.

In that final sermon that day, we had to reach back into
Matthew's Gospel for the actual story of Christ's transfiguration because John's Gospel doesn't include it. Why? Perhaps
because John's entire story is one of transfiguration, a story
about the stretching thin of those boundaries between us
and God, a story about the invisible being made visible in
the flesh, blood, words, and ministry of Jesus, a story about
where and how and through whom the very presence of
God is revealed to the likes of us—from Jesus first showing
up on the scene with John the Baptist, to his miraculous
signs, to his crucifixion on the cross, right through to his

very resurrection and appearance before grief-stricken and newly blind disciples who can't see what's right in front of their faces. Whatever it is that we might believe or not believe about Jesus, whatever it is that the world might say about who Jesus is or isn't, the transfiguration story gives us a glimpse behind the mask of Jesus's flesh and blood, that we might see the very presence of God in him and thus might also come to see that very presence of God through Jesus when our lives intersect with his presence.

Thus, I proclaimed to my flock:

If—and it's a big "if"—*if* there is anything to the positive that cancer has done to me, it is to further thin out those boundaries between the seen and unseen in my life. Even on the days that are less than ideal. Even on the days that have been racked with pain or other side effects—and those have become blessedly fewer and further in between for now. Even on the days that have become, thankfully, normal and uneventful. Even on the days that I am tied up in insurance company hell. Every last one of them is a day in which I, through the waters of baptism, have been promised Christ's presence. And every last one of these days become days where faith invites me not only to hope for that presence, but to see it and to bear witness to it.

And from there, I named some of the moments, ways, and places I had witnessed God's grace in the steadfast presence of Kari and the kids; in the overflowing freezer full of meals folks had delivered; in the intervention my oncologist had provided when the insurance company refused coverage for a needed drug; in the devices that allowed Karl and me and our people to stay in touch in spite of my treatments and Karl's monthlong hospitalization following his diagnosis.

I concluded the sermon, literally overcome and a blubbering mess with emotion, from the standpoint of both the overwhelming power of Christ's realized and received promises and the grief and uncertainty about how this ordeal would end, for me, my family, and my congregation:

> The stories of Scripture—the Word of God—aren't just stories "about" Jesus. They are also stories that create faith and hope and the ability to see Jesus not just in the written and proclaimed word, but in our very lives, as well, especially when we labor under the crosses we bear. Christ is there in the midst of our suffering, giving us what we ourselves lack, to see, to believe, to worship, and to be borne up in our suffering.

Whatever the impact of those words on my listeners, they were words I needed to hear.

Throughout my treatments, our mailbox and front steps continually received cards, well-wishes, and gifts, the "Cheetos" that communicated not just the thoughts and prayers of friends, family, and parishioners but their "presence," even if they couldn't literally "go," as Rolf's lesson encourages. The week after my final sermon leading into my temporary medical disability leave, a particularly large Amazon box appeared on our front step, and in that box was an entire case of single-serving bags of Cheetos, a three-pound bag of Jolly Rancher hard candies, and this note:

> Even though we can't be with you, we want you to know we love you. Enjoy the Cheetos. Eric found Jolly Ranchers

to be particularly helpful for warding off the bad tastes that came with his chemo. Eric, Jackie, Allison, Brody, and Connor.

Let those with ears hear.

————————

### KARL (2022)

To a certain degree this whole cancer thing wasn't my first rodeo, having lived it alongside Rolf back in the '80s. But in my wife's case this was far more pointedly so. Angela lost her first husband, Rick Fairbanks, to pancreatic cancer. She'd been down this road before, to the worst possible degree. One of the great insights she shared was that, at a certain point, she just couldn't take any more questions, even questions like, "What do you need?" or "How can I help?" Believe it or not, those kinds of questions can, for some people, ramp up the stress levels. What Angela came to realize was that when someone offered something specific, it actually relieved the stress. What was most helpful for Angela (and so for me too) were things like this:

> "Can I swing by and weed your garden for you?" (Yes, weeding had definitely gone by the wayside.)
>
> "I'm a handyman. Does anything around your house need fixing?" (Have you met Karl, the world's second-least-handy man? [Have you met Rolf?] Yes, some things needed fixing.)
>
> "I make a mean cheesecake. Let me make you one for Easter." (Yes, yes, a thousand times yes!)

Here's the thing. When someone you care about is suffering, and there is nothing you can say or do to make cancer go away, or the unknown known, when you can't "fix it," you can "fix stuff." Offer to do what you love to do or are good at; offer your*self* and share in people's suffering that way. You can't "fix" things, but *you* can fix things. You can make things better, more hopeful, more bearable by showing up.

---

People are helpers, and people are fixers. These are two of the most wonderful things about human nature. When a loved one is suffering, people want to help the suffering one, and people want to fix the cause of suffering. And here, either things can go a little bit sour, or (by the grace of God) things can go miraculously sweet. At the risk of coming off a little bit grandiose, we want to offer some rules about caring for someone who is suffering.

*Caregiving Rule 1: Understand that "hurt people hurt people."*[5] Someone who has been hurt is quite likely to hurt others in ways similar to, or stemming from, how they have been hurt. If you are caring for someone who has been hurt or is suffering, that person may express anger—and from time to time you might be on the receiving end. They may lash out. They may shout. They might wind up into themselves like a coil and then spring out in their pain. *Ordinary People* is a novel by Judith Guest, which was made into a movie by the same title, starring Mary Tyler Moore.[6] The plot of *Ordinary People* revolves around how a father (Calvin), mother (Beth), and younger son (Conrad) cope with their pain following the accidental death of the family's older son (Buck). As the story unfolds, the three surviving members of the family hurt each other in subtle but deeply harmful ways. Finally, Beth, unable to live in the same household with Calvin, Conrad, and her own pain, leaves the family. But Calvin and Conrad are able to lean on each other by leaning into each other's pain.

We have two bits of wisdom about offering care and love to those who are lashing out in the midst of their suffering. First, it is often the case that people in pain lash out at those whom they love and trust the most (spouses, parents, siblings, friends), or at those in positions of authority (pastors, counselors, teachers, and ultimately God). If you find yourself on the receiving end of the anger or pain of someone who is suffering, try to think of it as a compliment. Tell yourself something like, "Hey, my son is angry with me for no fault of my own, or for something that I didn't do. He really trusts me." Or, "My wife just really dressed me down, and all I did was put the toilet paper roll on backward. She still loves me as much as ever." This can be very hard to do in the moment when you are on the short end of the stick, but it is a very helpful coping technique—and it has the virtue of also being true.

Second—and this may seem a little abstract—don't run from the pain, but rather lean into the pain. Lean into the pain you are experiencing, and lean into the pain of the suffering one. For pretty obvious reasons, human beings don't like pain. Biologically, pain is a signal that something is wrong. Pain may be telling us that there is something dangerous that needs to be avoided, such as fire or extreme cold. In these cases, pain may be a signal to avoid the fire, to avoid the freezing cold. But sometimes pain might be telling us that there is something wrong that needs to be healed, such as when a person has a cut or an infection. In this case, the pain is a signal to attend to the cut or the infection. Deep emotional, psychological, and spiritual pain is like this. One cannot flee from it or avoid it, because it lies deep inside of us. If we try to avoid it, or deny it, or numb it, the root cause of the pain might grow worse. If we try to numb the pain with alcohol, drugs, or some other tactic of denial, the root cause might not go away, and we might develop a secondary problem—alcoholism or chemical dependency.

To "lean into the pain" means to face it, to name a painful situation for what it is and accept that it hurts. To lean into the pain means we are not going to ignore it, deny it, or numb it. And when we do this together, we can face most pain. This is even more true when we learn to invite God into our pain and lean into the pain of the Holy One who endured the cross on our behalf. The same is true of fear. Fear is natural, and fear of things—of danger, of getting hurt, of the dark, of there being strawberry in the rhubarb pie—serves a purpose. So name the fear, own it, don't try to dispel it. And don't let it own you.

*Caregiving Rule 2: Giving care is about what to say and do when nothing you can say or do can fix the root problem.* Think back to the story of the book of Job. Job had lost everything. Because his friends loved him, they came to see him and sit with him in his pain. Because they could see that his pain was very great, they didn't say anything. What a good and wise decision! But later, they couldn't help themselves, and they just had to talk.

Sometimes, a crisis or tragedy hits, and there is nothing that you can do to address the underlying reality—such as when a loved one develops cancer, or when a loved one dies, or when one's parents divorce, or when one is seriously injured in an accident, or when one loses one's home. We could multiply the examples, but you get the point. When crises arise we may be inclined to bury our heads in the sand, either to avoid facing our own suffering, or so that we don't have to see the suffering of those we love. Our calling as people of faith, hope, and love is to go there anyway, even though we can't fix the situation. As caregivers, we have the privilege—and yes, it is a privilege—to enter into the crisis and stand with the one who is facing it.

People are fixers by nature. When a diagnosis such as cancer arrives, people want to help. So they try to figure out what they can do to help. Some of our friends researched what was the best hospital for sarcoma, or leukemia, or lymphoma. They researched what the newest medical treatments are for those cancers. Some of our friends researched non-Western treatments for our cancers. Other friends preached the glories and wonders of various diets: "Have you tried vegan?" Or, "A Paleo diet might be the best response to chemotherapy." Or, "Intermittent fasting worked for me when I had cancer." And so on.

When Rolf was fighting cancer in high school, a professional football player whose NFL career had been derailed by injury called Rolf. He had never met Rolf but heard about Rolf's story from a mutual acquaintance. In an effort to get his career back on track, he was driving to Texas for a faith-healing event and offered to take Rolf with him. People want to help; we are fixers by nature. Other friends, recognizing that Rolf's primary hobbies and pastimes were now gone— tennis, skiing, marching band—brought well-intentioned gifts. One friend gave him an art kit (Rolf has absolutely no artistic talent).

But sometimes, there is nothing we can do to address the underlying problem. But this doesn't mean we can't do anything! Rather, it means recognizing what we can and cannot do. The second rule of caring for those in crisis is to *recognize when we can meaningfully help the underlying crisis and when we cannot.* Or rather, it means recognizing that most of the time we cannot do anything meaningful about the underlying crisis.

In these situations, the key is—as we like to say—to do three things. First, show up. Second, say, "I love you. I'm sorry that this is happening. It's awful. And I love you." Third, bring Cheetos. Because, after all, Cheetos are the perfect way to say, "I love you." Or, bring a game. Bring a bottle of scotch. Bring cheese. Bring something that says, "I love you."

*Caregiving Rule 3: Stick with it.* All too often, when the dust settles people move on, and they aren't aware of the after-effects and the struggles that may be ongoing, struggles that are physical, emotional, and spiritual. Even when things seem to be finished, or on the upswing, the stresses and the pain can still be there. This is most obvious, perhaps, when someone suffers the death of a loved one. After time has passed, the loss may fade for others, but still it remains. So stick with it; don't stop the caregiving.

One simple way to do this is to mark anniversaries, even anniversaries of things we certainly aren't celebrating. On the morning of February 17, 2021, after the alarm clock had been silenced, Karl's wife Angela rolled over and said, "Happy anniversary." The point was not, "Hey, remember that great day when you were diagnosed with leukemia?" The point was, "Here we are, a year later. We've got this." Stick with it. Mark the milestones. Stay connected. Don't forget. Stay faithful.

*Caregiving Rule 4: No one is perfect.* Do not be too hard on yourself. You won't be perfect. We have not been perfect—not in caring for ourselves, not in caring for each other, and not in caring for other friends and neighbors.

———

## KARL (2010)

Here's the thing: No one is perfect. We are talking about how to do this caregiving thing, and I, for one, have to confess that I haven't always been able to do it. In the early 2000s one of my oldest and closest friends, Anthony Simione, was battling a benign brain tumor ("benign," which means "gentle," or "kindly"—which tells you all you need to know about medical terminology). He had had surgery and was living well with the disease—with complications, for sure, but well. But it kept coming back, and in the end turned cancerous; he was terribly compromised. And the truth of the matter is that I wasn't the faithful friend to him that I wish I could have been. I had my reasons, having to do with family issues that it's not worth getting specific about, but no excuses. In the first days of his recovery from brain surgery I had visited him in the hospital and spent time with him. I bought him Lego sets so that he could rehone his fine motor skills. But, over time, my availability for him lessened. In his last year we went to a movie once (2010's *A-Team*), and in his very last days I sat with him and held his hand when he was mostly unresponsive. But that was about it.

I didn't show up in the way I wish I had for a friend I'd gone to grade school, junior high, and high school (sort of) with, and with whom I roomed three out of four years in college. I didn't show up for his wife, Stephanie, who had been a friend for almost twenty years. I didn't show up for his kids, who were the same age as my own. I didn't show up for his parents, who had been mentors and caregivers to me since childhood. It would have been easy for Stephanie (and others) to shut me out after that. But she didn't. Her graciousness and understanding have been one of the great gifts of any friendship I've had. Over time, we've been able to share memories and joys, as well as regrets and sorrows, in ways that have been healing for me, and, I trust, helpful for her as well. So, once again, it's never too late.

This needs to be said: No one is perfect. Least of all me. (Well, least of all the apostle Paul, who described himself as "the foremost" of sinners [1 Tim. 1:15].) You aren't perfect. But you don't have to be. And it doesn't take much to make it right—just humility, grace, and faithfulness.

---

### ROLF (NOVEMBER 1990)

On the ten-year anniversary of my cancer diagnosis, I was a senior in seminary, in St. Paul, Minnesota. At the time, my parents were living in Iowa. My sister Karen was living in Rochester, Minnesota, while my sister Anne and her new husband, Bill, were living in Madison, Wisconsin. Our friends Jerry and Jean Larson were still living in Northfield. I called my dad and asked if we could mark the anniversary of my cancer by eating at the Fisherman's Inn outside of Rochester, and I wondered if we could invite Jerry and Jean to join us. (My brother, Karl, was in China at the time, so he missed out on this dinner. But don't worry, he probably was eating his favorite food—some delicious and authentic Chinese dumpling. He was happy.)

So, it was arranged. On the ten-year anniversary of cancer and initial amputation, my family and the Larsons converged on the Fisherman's Inn.

At the time, I had a new girlfriend, who had not yet met any of my family and who did not yet know the full story of my cancer. I picked her up, and we began the seventy-five-minute drive.

She asked, "I'm looking forward to dinner and meeting your family, but can you tell me why we are going to this restaurant?"

I answered, "Well, at the worst part of the worst part of my war with cancer, my dad's friend Jerry dragged me to dinner at this place. When we got there, he asked the waitress, 'How are your ribs?'"

In the more than forty years since my original diagnosis, I have learned the importance of marking anniversaries and celebrating milestones. My friends in recovery celebrate the anniversaries of their sobriety. My friends who are military veterans commemorate the anniversaries of their service, or key battles, or their military units. Many of my friends mark the anniversaries of a loved one's death. And so on. I celebrate the years of my survival, the years since my last surgery, and other key moments along the way.

I have learned that these anniversaries are important. In the early years, I would want to be alone or just get together with a close friend or two. Such anniversaries are a chance to give thanks to God for life, to remember the bad times and the good times, to recall all of the people who helped me get through it. These are good things to do: Be sad, be happy, remember, be grateful, recollect, reminisce, recoil, wince, cry, thank God.

There isn't a right way to celebrate these anniversaries. Some people go on trips. Or go skydiving. Some people get away for a break or go on a silence retreat. Others have friends over.

I eat ribs.

On that ten-year anniversary date, we all arrived at the Fisherman's Inn. Here's a funny thing about that evening. In the nine years since the original night when Jerry, Dad, and I ate at that restaurant (which happened one year into my battle with cancer), I never once talked with Jerry about that meal. I never thanked him or told him how much that evening meant to me. I never told him how much I appreciated that bright moment of light during the darkest time of my life.

But Jerry must have known. Or, at the very least, when we invited him back to the same restaurant nine years later, he must have remembered.

We all took our seats at the table. Mom and Dad, Jerry and Jean, Anne and Bill, Karen, me and my new girlfriend. We ordered our drinks. The waitress asked if we had any questions about the menu.

And Jerry said, "How are your ribs?"

Without a cue, just as he did nine years before that, he put on the whole show. "I'm not getting through to you!" "Your favorite uncle is coming to town!" "His favorite food is ribs!" "Would you let him eat your ribs?" The whole show.

And then he picked up the check.

> You prepare a table before me
>     in the presence of my enemies;
> you anoint my head with oil;
>     my cup overflows. (Ps. 23:5)

87

# 4

# Laughter

## Finding Joy in the Midst of Illness and Disability

The righteous will see, and fear, and will laugh.
—Psalm 52:6a

Strength and dignity are her clothing,
and she laughs at the time to come.
—Proverbs 31:25

Stand-up comedian and actor Robert Klein once shared this: "People ask me, 'Is there anything that's off limits?' No, but if you do a joke about cancer, it better be funny."[1]

Time for a bit of a confession, in case you haven't picked up on it by now: All three of us think most everything is funny. Or at least that there can be something funny or humorous in pretty much anything, even the hardest things.

89

What's more, humor is an essential means of "changing the temperature"—of reshaping mood, yes, but of doing far more than that.

We believe that it is not only possible but essential to find joy, laughter, and abundant life in the midst of suffering, illness, and disability.

In his 2007 book *Religious Literacy*,[2] Stephen Prothero offered a basic test of religious literacy with questions asking readers if they could list the four biblical Gospels, what the first five books of the Old Testament are, what the First Amendment of the Constitution says about religion, and so on.[3] He also asked whether this is true or false: "'God helps he who helps himself' is in the Bible." (The answer, if you don't know, is false.) Another such question he might have asked is, True or false: "Laughter is the best medicine" is in the Bible? And the answer might surprise you, because it's true. Well, at least sort of true. Proverbs 17:22 says this:

> A cheerful heart is a good medicine,
>   but a downcast spirit dries up the bones.

This biblical proverb is often cited as the origin for the modern proverb, "Laughter is the best medicine." Maybe, maybe not, but here is the point that both of these proverbs are making: Good cheer and joy, good humor and laughter help us. We would go a step further and say that laughter is a spiritual gift.

God's Easter promise is that death has been defeated and the future life of the creation has been assured. Death will not have the last word, because its sting has been pulled (1 Cor. 15:51–56). Creation will not die—there will be a new creation. As Paul writes, "So if anyone is in Christ, there is a new creation: everything old has passed away; see, everything has become new!" (2 Cor. 5:17). Laughter and joy are spiritual gifts because they are ways of receiving God's Easter promise. The very nature of the good news—the gospel—is that it is *promise*. Not just a promise, but divine promise itself. And faith is receiving, believing, trusting, and living in that promise as if it were true. The promise: Your sins are forgiven. Trust is accepting forgiveness and forgiving one another. The sacramental promise: I am with you. Faith is believing that God is with us and that God's new creation will break into being all around us. The baptismal promise: You are mine; I know you, I have called you by name, and I love you. Faith is knowing whose we are and who loves us, and loving all who are loved by God. The Easter promise: Death is defeated; it has no sting—eternal and abundant life are ours. Faith is living God's gift of abundant life in the Spirit right now. Faith is laughing in the face of death because death has been defeated! Even though we are still living in the midst of suffering, illness, and disability. When we laugh in the midst of cancer, it is a way of receiving the promise of new life. When we laugh in the midst of disability, it is a way of receiving the promise of new creation. When we laugh in the midst of pain, it is a way of receiving the promise that Christ will wipe away every tear and that there will be no more weeping.

---

## MIKE (2022)

When I first shared these thoughts through my CaringBridge blog, I prefaced them with this warning: "These observations may not be for those who tend to shy away from open talk about bodily functions and privacy." Not everyone shares the same "inappropriate," even gallows, humor in which my closest friends, my family, and I found comfort and relief from the pain that cancer brings. Interestingly enough, the most common response I got from those kinds of blog entries were things like, "I have found your openness and humor toward these things refreshing."

One of the memories I had of my father-in-law's bout with colon cancer twenty-plus years ago was his observation—one that I now share—that privacy and bodily modesty are *out the window* when it comes to cancer treatment. I suspect that this is true of medical treatment and hospital life in general, as well. There comes a point with the body and its treatment when it begins to feel like my body doesn't belong just to me anymore. (And I think there's some theology, some God-talk, cooking in that statement.)

This takes *a lot* of getting used to, especially, I think, if one has or has had body confidence issues or body insecurity issues to begin with. Likewise, perhaps, if you've been raised in a demure, modest, and private sort of way about the body and its functions. It really had been only over the last year of exercise and intentional wellness that I had gotten reacclimated to mine.

Early on, even just the request to undress—"You can leave your underwear on. [Why, thank you!] And here's a 'gown' [half a gown, anyway] to put on"—felt weird the first time I heard it. And that wasn't just the breeze up the backside.

As was recounted in chapter 1, when I had my first contrast dye CT scan to uncover the extent of the cancer, the tech told me, "You might experience one of the strangest

92

sensations you've ever felt, which will begin with a not-so-unpleasant warmth beginning at your shoulders, culminating with that warmth around your behind." I discovered the reality of the matter was that she really didn't mean my "behind," as in the gluteus muscles in my butt. There was a deeper, smaller, specific part of the plumbing involved. When I had my second contrast dye CT scan, the tech began to give me a similar warning. "Oh, I know where this is headed," I told her. If you know, you know (or, as the kids abbreviate it: IYKYK). And this was the handy piece of information I shared with Karl as he anticipated the same procedure and we shared a laugh about together once it was complete.

Next, the poking and prodding by people you hardly know in places that only a few choice people have ever even had access to is jarring and unsettling. Fart jokes are one thing at the Pancoastmania dinner table—I will probably always have an inner fourteen-year-old to contend with—but it's a whole other thing when a stranger, even in a clinical setting, is so concerned about your bowels, your consistency, and your urine output and color. Even to have someone who isn't my wife come in and help me get my T-shirt over my head and up my chemo tubing and IV tower just to have a shower is humbling, if not humiliating. And it isn't anything remotely sexualized at all—just a sense of pathos that this body is an open book to all these people whose mission it is to heal me and make me well. One will struggle mightily if one isn't able to find some laughter in those ordeals.

I found myself oversharing a lot when people asked me how I was doing. My response was: "Do you really want to know? Because I *will* tell you."

I think the open book of my body led to an open book of my heart, mind, and mouth, as well. And while the laughter around such things was probably off-putting to some, it also lowered the defense mechanisms of propriety behind which we often hide in uncomfortable situations. I think what I came to realize in the absurdity of cancer and the loss of privacy is that we aren't just bodies. Furthermore, these human bodies in which we exist by the Creator's intent are wondrous, ridiculous things. This is especially true of the less delicate aspects of those bodies, their plumbing, and their ventilation! But my well-being, my health, my healing and wellness aren't just tied up with bodily functions and symptoms or the lack thereof but are found also in my mental attitude and faith and spirituality. And those of us who are followers of Jesus, the incarnate Son of God, follow him as the revelation of God in flesh and blood. Because this is true, we must learn to experience God's grace in real, tangible ways in the warp and woof of life, *including in and through our bodies*. (I found myself at times marveling at the thought that Jesus himself had in his humanity the exact same body parts and functions as me!)

Maybe this is all a little bit TMI—too much information. But my tendency to overshare isn't intended to be off-putting, offensive, or awkward—though admittedly, I suppose, it likely had that effect for some. For me, I think there were two things going on.

First, the search for homeostasis, stability, and equilibrium in a time that was anything but stable for me produced a lot of humor and laughter over the absurdity of all this. Good comedy is sometimes a quest for working things out, literally, from the inside out—topics and thoughts that are so strange that we have to laugh, lest we cry. I don't know if I was doing good comedy or not, but I was definitely trying to make others laugh by sharing, and I was trying to assure them that I was as okay as I could be by getting them to laugh with and even at me: "Rejoice with me, and sing, for I have given two and a half fully formed bowel movements over the last three days!" Or, one of my favorites at the hospital was in response to the question of whether I was passing gas: "Like a *champ!*" (Like I said, I will probably always have to contend with an inner fourteen-year-old.)

The second thing I think I became aware of in all of this body talk was a fear of being alone in my situation. I needed my closest people to be able to share with me both the humor and, once again, the humiliating pathos that it masked. "Maybe that's you," I wrote on CaringBridge. "And maybe it's not. Which is perfectly OK." But that thought— "Don't be surprised if you ask how I am, and I ask you, 'Do you really want to know?' because I will tell you"—became an invitation to meet me where I was. The intent was not to embarrass people. The intent was to invite them to be a part of what I was going through, so that I was not alone in the absurdity of my body and what it was going through. In laughing together, I could be as well as I could be.

In June of 2022, toward the end of my treatment, I was receiving high doses of a chemo drug called methotrexate, intended to be an insurance policy against recurrence. That treatment featured taking what were essentially baking soda pills at home beginning the Sunday morning before Monday's in-hospital admission in order to bring my body's pH to 7.5 to 8.0—remember your high school chemistry: pH is the measure of a solution's acidity (less than 7) or basicity (higher than 7)—in order to protect my kidneys for what was about to happen to them. A quick round of blood work at the cancer center, a visit with the oncologist and care coordinating nurse (who was *fabulous*!), and then we'd be off to be admitted at St. Cloud Hospital.

Occasionally I got the question from folks, "So, is this chemo harder or easier than your previous cycles?" I'd say, "I don't get sick from this at all, but the process is considerably more putzy." Here's what that meant: Apparently, the only way to test my body's pH is the urine. So when I'd get to the hospital, in addition to the handfuls of baking soda tablets every four hours, I would also get hooked up to a huge bag of sodium bicarbonate solution *and* was encouraged to drink *lots* of water—quarts and quarts of water. Would that I could've just licked a pH paper strip, because what *really* would happen is that I had to pee into a bottle; call one of the staff, who then had to take a sample from the bottle to send down to the lab; and then we would wait to make sure my pH was where it was supposed to be. And this had to happen every . . . single . . . hour. Every single hour some poor soul would have to come and deal with my pee.

But wait! There's more!

After my body's pH reached 7.5, next came the methotrexate, which looked like Mountain Dew. Unlike the R-EPOCH chemo, which was infused at a constant rate over twenty-four hours, Monday through Friday, the methotrexate only took an hour or so.

But then the peeing *really* began. Because in order for me to go home, the methotrexate level in my blood had to reach 0.1 or lower. Twenty-four hours after the methotrexate had been administered, next I would get a drug infusion called leucovorin that protected my kidneys from the high dose methotrexate, and lots and lots and *lots* of water. And the whole process continued: Pee in the bottle; call one of the staff to come grab the sample and measure the amount of my "output"; and then wait for the lab to send the results of *both* my pH *and* the methotrexate.

"Expect three to four days in the hospital" was the guidance of the oncologist and care coordinating nurse. In on Monday. Out by Wednesday or Thursday.

In all of those final cycles, I was able to complete them in as little as two and a half days, earning me the reputation as—at least, according to my favorite nurse, Caleb—"The fastest pee-er I've ever seen!"

In the words of Larry the Cable Guy, "That there's funny. I don't care who you are."

----

## KARL (2022)

There were, for me, lots of ways in which humor changed things for me, both while I was hospitalized and while I was recovering from the bone marrow transplant (BMT). My oldest child, Thursday, came to visit me in the early days of my first hospital stay. I'd already started chemotherapy, and because of the leukemia my blood wasn't clotting the way it's supposed to. As a result, when I had my first bone marrow biopsy I ended up with a massive hematoma (subdural bleeding; think big, ugly bruise) that ran from my right hip all the way down to my calf. It wasn't pretty. *I* wasn't pretty. And it hurt a lot. In fact, that was the most physically painful part of my entire experience. Thursday walked in, saw me laid out in my hospital bed and gown, and said, "You look like crap." Is that any way to talk to your father?! Is that any way to talk to your father who just had a leukemia diagnosis?! Outrageous behavior! Insult to injury! And, absolutely classic, genuine Thursday. It made me laugh, and it brightened my day.

As I was about to go in for my transplant, once again my friend Greg came through. He sent me a daily calendar called "You Had One Job." The product description goes like this: "This daily desktop calendar features some of the all-time funniest, most ridiculous workplace blunders that will leave you laughing, crying, and exclaiming, 'You had one job!'" I had that calendar with me in the hospital and during my seventy days of isolation at home. In an almost ritualistic sense I looked forward to reading the blunder of the day, usually right after breakfast, and getting a chuckle out of it. Embracing that humor was as much a part of my day as prayer.

One of the side effects of a BMT is that your childhood vaccinations are nullified, and so about a year later you have to get all of those shots all over again. When I went in to get the first series of shots, I was given a vaccine information sheet, so I'd know what to expect. The funny thing was they didn't bother to write up a sheet specifically for adults, so the fact sheet read, "Your Child's First Vaccines: What You Need to Know." I was a toddler again! (Okay, let's be honest, *still*.) And the first thing on the list of what to expect? Fussiness. I took full advantage of that, let me tell you.

For my own part, finding the ridiculous, the silly, and the laughter in all of it helped me to face everything that was in front of me. Here's one example.

## CaringBridge Entry | June 8, 2022[4]

What is the worst part of this cancer thing? It's simple: all the math. Which of my chromosomes are mutated, p210 or p190? (Apparently neither number is better or worse, nor does it matter in terms of the treatment plan, so why use numbers at all?) How many different medications will I be on? Like twelve. Pills per day? Upward of thirty.

There are so many numbers flying around and at us that I can't help but think of two of Saturday Night Live's presidential impersonations: Chevy Chase's Gerald Ford saying, "It was my understanding that there would be no math," and Will Ferrell's George Bush, who said, "Math, which is also part of the axis of evil."

Math is, as my nephew Gunnar might have said as a little boy, "Yuck," which is why at St. Olaf for my math requirement I took a course called "Math for Poets." (I'll never forget the opening line of the course description: What does math mean to the sunflower?) Math; as a rule, I've tried to avoid it. But there are, alas, lots and lots of numbers in my life these days.

112 days since my original diagnosis.

28 days at Regions Hospital before going home.

7 days back in the hospital with a fever.

"First remission" for the past 22 days.

Tomorrow will be day -5 of the bone marrow transplant process [i.e., five days until surgery].

Today was the second day of my sister's bone marrow harvesting.

She is giving at the rate of 5 million cells per kilogram of my weight, which for you nosy types is about 97.5224 kilograms (which you can multiply by 2.2 to find my weight in pounds), so overall that's something like 487,612,000 in total. (Have you ever had someone give you 487 million of something?! I sure hope I have room.)

On days -4 to -1 I will have twice-daily, full-body radiation treatments that will last about 20 minutes each. This is to prep me to receive the 487 million gifts coming my way by way of transfusion on day 0. Day 0, which really makes no kind of sense; shouldn't it be day 1?

Anyway, after day 0 I will have 3–5 weeks of inpatient care at the U of M Medical Center.

If all goes well, I will then be discharged to fill out the rest of the 100 days of "close care," during which I cannot be more than 30 minutes from the hospital, in the case that my body decides to return the gifts given (yes, I'll save the receipt).

During those 70-odd days at home I will need 24/7 close care—that's right, I can't be left unsupervised and *yes*, that *is* a change from before cancer, thank you very much—by folks 18 years and older with a license to drive.

After those 100 days it will likely be another 3–6 months before I'm ready to be back in the swing of "normal" life.

Some other *real* numbers. The BMT is the only cure for this leukemia, but it is dangerous as well. There is a 75–80 percent survival rate, and so a 20–25 percent mortality rate after the transplant. This may sound scary, but as my son, Sam, said, "At least the survival rate isn't 2 percent." And that's right.

Some other numbers from along the way:

A year of full-time disability is covered by our fine health insurance, at two-thirds of regular income, which kind of stinks, but on the upside I'm not driving much these days, so not having to fill up at $4.64 per gallon (as of June 8th) is making a huge difference.

2 trips to the cabin with my dad.

1 with my brother.

1 with my kids, Thursday, Sam, and Lucy.

3 largemouth bass caught (and released, because, while I didn't want to eat them, I *did* want to make them late for something—thanks for that joke, Mitch Hedberg) by me.

2 fish caught by Lucy.

0 fish caught by my brother (loser).

2 years ago June 9th was our dog Moses's adoption day.

1 year ago it was move-in day for us into our new home.

And, lastly, countless are God's mercies, and the prayers said for us; and immeasurable the love that we are feeling from so many of you.

Thanks, as always, for reading and chiming in as you are moved; those responses lift us up.

When cancer comes calling, or suffering threatens to overwhelm you, embrace humor as God's gift to help you through it. Laugh. Laugh at illness; laugh at "the evildoer"; laugh at death, even; laugh at (read: because of) Christ's faithfulness on the cross, and in death, and in resurrection. Laugh with God the great Easter laugh. Laughter and joy in the face of disability, illness, suffering, and even death are a way of receiving God's Easter promise and living in faith.

––––––––

## ROLF (1989 . . . AND A LOT OF OTHER YEARS)

Here's the deal: If you are going to live with no legs, spending most of the day in a wheelchair, you had better learn to laugh

101

at your yourself, learn to laugh at the absurdities that come with life in a disabled body, and learn to embrace the delightful absurdities that abound all around. The alternatives are either that you boil away in anger or that you wrap yourself in numbness. I can't recommend either of those alternatives, so I have chosen to laugh at as much of life as I can. There are lots of examples, but I will start with my favorite and offer a few more.

In 1989, while I was in seminary, I moved west to serve my internship in Mount Vernon, Washington—a delightful town with much to recommend it: mountains, mild winters and summers, Puget Sound, and entire fields of tulips in the spring. In other words, nothing like Minnesota.

One of my first stops in Mount Vernon was the local Target. While I was there, I heard a kid behind me say to his father, "Hey, Dad! Look! Someone's wearing a bike!"

You know what? That's pretty funny. In my forty plus years in a wheelchair, I've heard kids say some pretty unfiltered things about me. "Look, Mom! No legs!" is a pretty standard blurtation. I love the kids who come up and ask, "Hey, where are your legs?" I answer, "I don't have any legs." Small children will then usually ask, "Well, how do you get dressed?" (My mom explained to me that getting dressed by one's self is one of the milestones toward independence. So this odd-sounding question is really pretty perceptive— kids are really trying to put together a picture of how I can be independent while still having a disability.) I usually answer, "I put on my pants the same way you do . . . one stump at a time." Okay, that's not really true. Even I am not *that* mean. I used to answer, "It's easy!" Until one child got a sad look on his face and said, "I can't do it." So now

I answer, "After I lost my legs, I had to learn to get dressed again, but I learned."

When I tell kids, "I don't have any legs," some of the more curious want to know where they are. Some children smile as if I'm telling them a joke and ask, "Okay, where are they *really*?" Some of them get down and look under my wheelchair or look behind me. One kid said, "I bet they're in your car." When I tell kids that the doctors had to cut off my legs to save my life, many will ask, "What did they do with them after they cut them off?" At this point, I usually refrain from teaching a new phrase: "medical waste incinerator."

My favorite kid response of all time was the boy who said, "Someone's wearing a bike!" That seems like the most poetic description I've ever heard of what it's like to live in a wheelchair. I like it so much that I use it as part of my official biography: Rolf "generally wears a bicycle and a smile."

It was hard for my children—Ingrid and Gunnar—to get used to how people treat me. When we go out to a mall or restaurant, people stare at me. I don't notice anymore, but my kids do, and they had a really hard time with it, especially when they were in grade school. "Dad, people are staring." "Yeah," I would say, "I don't notice it anymore. When you are this beautiful, you have to get used to people staring."

It helps if you can learn to laugh at life. And sometimes you have to make your own laughs.

When I was in college, I loved to cheer on the sports teams. I had friends on the basketball team and would cheer them on from the stands behind the basket. When an opposing player toed the line to take a free throw, two football players (both named Jim) would lift me up—two arms but no legs—and shake me like a rag doll. They waved me back and forth, trying to distract the opposing player as he took aim for his free throws. (I learned about four years later that the ploy worked: I was a youth director at a church. One of the kids in the youth group attended a Christian school, and they had a chapel talk one day from a former varsity basketball player about "distractions in the Christian life." And he told a story about this kid with no legs. Hey! I never made varsity in sports, but I contributed to the team!)

With forty years of experience, I could tell stories all day long. But you get the point. Laugh at cancer. Laugh at disability. Laugh at death, even. It's a lot healthier than anger or numbness.

Learning to laugh at one's self and to laugh at the absurdities of life is another really good life hack. Humor and laughter got each of us through some pretty dismal times. Above all, if you have a choice between anger and humor, choose humor. In 2024, the comedian Jerry Seinfeld was granted an honorary degree by Duke University and invited to address the graduates at commencement. Seinfeld urged the graduates, "And this is probably the biggest point I would like to make to you here today, regarding humor . . . do not lose your sense of humor." He went on:

> You can have no idea at this point in your life how much you are going to need it to get through. Not enough of life makes sense for you to be able to survive it without humor. And I know all of you here are going to use all of your brains and muscle and soul to improve the world, and I know that you're going to do a bang-up job. And when you are done, as I am now, I bet the world, because of you, will be a much better place. But it will still not make a whole hell of a lot of

sense. It will be a better, different, but still pretty insane mess. And it is worth the sacrifice of an occasional discomfort to have some laughs. *Don't lose that.* Even if it's at the cost of occasional hard feelings, it's okay. You gotta laugh. That is the one thing at the end of your life you will not wish you did less of. *Humor is the most powerful, most survival-essential quality you will ever have or need to navigate through the human experience.*[5]

Humor allows us to face the most embarrassing moments and situations with grace. It helps other people overcome that uncomfortable feeling they might have around a sick person. It affords us the chance to create moments of joy and laughter in the middle of the crap.

Humor allows us to embrace life in its craziness, its absurdities, its ups and downs. But there is more to embracing life than just learning to laugh. You also need to learn to do hard things.

---

### ROLF (1983 AND 1994)

In order to embrace life with no legs and in a wheelchair, I needed to learn to do some hard things. And sometimes—maybe most of the time—I didn't and don't want to do hard things. I like easy things.

In April 1982, the doctors at Mayo Clinic amputated my remaining leg—thus ending the worst part of the worst part of my life. About two weeks later, my mom announced to me that it was time to go back to school. (In your imagination, insert silence and then a brooding soundtrack of growing doom.) It was the moment I was dreading. I would have to return to the hallways of high school with no legs. My mom told me that I would start by attending only the afternoon classes—which turned out to be German, French, and history. It was hard—seeing the pitying looks on classmates' faces and staring down academic subjects for which I had missed six months of classes.

But at home, my mom had my back and lent me some of her strength. And at school I had great friends—especially Jay Jasnoch, Jeff Streitz, Stefan Anderson, and Bernt Johnson—the kind of friends who would walk with you to Mordor if you had to dispose of a ring. It turns out that with family at your back and friends at your side, you can do hard things.

It was also time to return to church. And I was dreading returning to church. All of the church had been praying for me. The American Lutheran Church Women of our congregation had given me a television with a remote control when I was really, really sick. And I wasn't sure if I could hold it together emotionally if one of those wonderful women came up to me and said something caring or kind. So, being as devious as the Grinch, I would arrive for worship five minutes late and come in during the opening hymn. And I would leave at the start of the closing hymn. (Hey! Somebody had to get home and start making the gravy!)

But this was an avoidance response. And it couldn't go on forever. After two weeks, one Sunday morning my older sister Anne said, "I know what you are doing. Sooner or later, you are going to have to face people. How about we do it together today?" And we did. It turns out that with your big sister at your side, you can do hard things.

Over the years, many people helped me do hard things that I would never have believed that I could do. There are too many examples to count, but I want to relate three.

The first was in the winter of my senior year in high school. My two older sisters' favorite class in high school was German; and their favorite teacher was Herr Rockey. And so, my favorite class was German, with Herr Rockey. The pinnacle of the German curriculum was the senior-year trip to Germany. Starting sophomore year, Herr Rockey would show us slides of previous classes who made the trip, with many highlights. The castles of Mad King Ludwig—Hohenschwangau, where he grew up, and the three he built, Herrenchiemsee, Linderhof, and Neuschwanstein with its 350 stair steps. Up the mountain behind Neuschwanstein to the Marienbrucke. The salt mines of Berchtesgaden, where students would slide down a long salt shaft into the dark. The mountains—the unimposing Wank and the Zugspitze, the highest mountain in Germany. The fortified city of Rothenburg, with its circular wall and brick-and-cobbled streets. And the highlight, a weeklong stay with a German family. Sitting in my wheelchair—hearing about all of those steps, walls, mountains, chutes, ladders, and barriers—*I knew* that there was no way I could make that trip. There was no way.

One day after school, I was sitting in the computer room, focused on the monitor. A classmate named Gig Willson said, "Hi, Rolf, what are you doing?" I answered, "I'm playing on the computer." And I kept my focus on the computer. About ten or twenty seconds later he said, "Can we talk to you?" When I turned to look, I was surprised that Gig was not alone. A small group of my German class friends were with him. I'm not confident that I remember all of my classmates who were there. But I remember some of the faces—Gig, Stefan, Amy, Nathan, and Teri.

They said, "We saw that you didn't sign up for the trip to Germany. We are guessing that you aren't going because of what happened to you and because you're in a wheelchair. But we talked to Herr Rockey, and we want you to know that you are part of the class. We want you to go." At this point, one of my friends started to cry. "We will help you." That night, I talked to my parents about it. The next day, I talked to another classmate, Jay Jones. He said, "If you go, I'll help you. You can be my roommate." Suddenly, the trip that I had believed was impossible now seemed possible. It turns out that with friends at your side, you can do hard things.

The trip was the highlight of my high school years. My friends made it possible for me to go. They did so, first, by inviting and encouraging me. And second, by carrying me up all those steps (90 in Hohenschwangau and 350 in Neuschwanstein), up the mountain to the Marienbrucke, and all the rest. It wasn't easy for them—it was quite an imposition. But they helped and helped and never complained. Side note: In college, I majored in German and twice visited the family I met on the high school trip. Later, I returned with my wife and family twice. You really can do hard things with friends and family.

I would not blame you if you reflect back on my story and think, "Really? Going back to school, going to church, and going on a class trip!? Those were hard?! What adorable little first-world problems you have. Oh, little sweetie, do you need a teddy bear and a hug?"

If that's what you're thinking right now, you wouldn't be wrong. But those first, relatively minor "hard things" I had to do prepared me for the many harder things I would have to do later in life: going to college in a wheelchair; going to seminary (when I was not sure any congregation would hire a pastor with no legs); moving by myself to Mount Vernon, Washington, for a year of seminary internship at a church (the most important year of my education—thanks, Mark and Linda Johnson); taking a call as pastor at a church that was not handicapped accessible; buying my first car and my first house; earning my PhD in Old Testament; and most importantly, getting married and having kids. But the journey of ten thousand miles starts with one revolution of a wheelchair wheel, as the old saying goes. You have to do the first slightly hard thing in order to do all of the other, harder and harder things.

And you can do those hard things with family, friends, and God at your side. That is the true meaning of Paul's oft-quoted line, "I can do all things through him who strengthens me. In any case, it was kind of you to share my distress" (Phil. 4:13–14 NRSVue). Notice that Paul said he was able to do hard things with the help of God ("him who strengthens me") but also with the kind presence of those who shared in his difficult circumstances, his "distress." Because God has promised to be present in your life and promises to strengthen you, you can face the hard things that life throws in your way that you don't want to face. Because of the kind people around you who share in your distress, you are able to do all the things that you have to do.

# 5

# Survival

## Living in the Aftermath of Illness

.

I will extol you, O LORD, for you have drawn me up,
  and did not let my foes rejoice over me.
O LORD my God, I cried to you for help,
  and you have healed me.
O LORD, you brought up my soul from Sheol,
  restored me to life from among those gone down
    to the Pit.

—Psalm 30:1–3

————

**KARL (2022)**

When cancer comes calling, your whole world seems to be in turmoil; everything is upset, and there is no "normal." As soon as I was diagnosed with leukemia, the turmoil set in: I was immediately admitted to the hospital, my teenage girls

111

came home from school to an empty house (though my adult niece, Ingrid, was soon there), and my wife had to cut her sabbatical short and rush home from a retreat center in the Cascade mountains of Washington. Over the next days and months, we learned about the timing of it all: first, treatment to first remission; second, a bone marrow transplant; third, a lengthy period of recovery; fourth, a year or more to slowly build back strength. The uncertainty about what life after treatment might be raised questions. Would I ever return to full health and strength? Would I be able to return to full-time work? All of this was tumultuous, to say the least. But life went on, life *goes* on, in the midst of tumult.

As that first summer was coming to an end, my stepdaughter Nora was supposed to start her first year of college in Atlanta. The first year of college is a big deal—both for a child, whose collegiate life is about to begin, and also for a mother, whose firstborn is spreading her wings to leave the nest. Angela shared that Nora had asked if she should delay college so that she could stay home and help. Our answer was, "Absolutely not." Life must go on. Even in the midst of cancer treatments and recovery, day-to-day life matters.

Even as we write this book I am not all the way through the tumult. While I am currently in remission, my recovery of strength, energy, and stamina has been slow. In the run-up to the transplant, my doctor at the University of Minnesota Masonic Cancer Clinic, Joseph Maakaron, described how, generally, I could expect to do physically over time. He told me that after the transplant and the first one hundred days I would be at roughly 50 percent of my usual strength, energy, and stamina. After three to six months I would maybe be at 70 percent. And so on. At about the one-year mark posttransplant, I was making progress but felt that my recovery wasn't tracking, so during a checkup I asked Dr. Maakaron when I could expect to be back to 100 percent. Maakaron, who I think I'd seen smile twice in a year, barked out a laugh and said, "Karl, you'll never be 100 percent again. You're in your fifties, and you're a year older, so there's that. And we've done horrible things to your body. You'll need to get used to a new 100 percent."

I had to laugh. A "new" 100 percent, that will actually be less than 100 percent, at least the 100 percent I was used to. Again with the math. Life after disease will almost always be life with a "new normal." What that will look like, nobody knows, and in my case I am still figuring it out. But the blessing in all of this is that there *is* a new normal to be had. Life goes on, and I am grateful for the gift that this restored life can be.

There's an old truism that Winston Churchill most assuredly did *not* say (even though all kinds of folks claim he did), and that country music singer Rodney Atkins turned into an overly melodramatic and remarkably successful song in 2006, that goes like this: "If you're going through hell, don't stop." It's on target, if a little trite. This is one of the key lessons to be learned about facing cancer, or just about any other struggle: Don't stop.

Don't stop living daily life, don't stop the normal things, and above all, don't stop fighting. Fight and fight and fight, and, win, lose, or draw, don't stop. As Mike shares later in this chapter, using battle imagery drawn from Psalm 144 was helpful for him. Not every fight is a literal fight, and oftentimes martial imagery gets used in metaphorical ways that aren't helpful. But when cancer comes calling, no matter what kind of cancer it is, it's "fight night." It's like the great ring announcer Michael Buffer says, "Let's get ready to rumble!"

And here is, we hope, a life-giving insight: This fight against cancer isn't a "win, lose, or draw" scenario. Only two of those options are really in play. Norm Macdonald, in his standup set called "Me Doing Standup," told a joke about cancer. The joke is about an uncle who had cancer, and when he finally died, people were saying things like, "'He lost his battle.' That's no way to end your life, you know? What a loser that guy was. The last thing he did was lose." Macdonald then goes on to say, "I'm pretty sure, I'm not a doctor, but . . . I mean, if you die, the cancer also dies at exactly the same time, so that, to me, it's not a loss. That's a draw."

Win, or draw, that's the battle against cancer. And we would take it a step further. For the person of Christian faith, even death is not ultimately a loss—because Christ has already given us victory over the grave. That is not to say that there isn't real loss, or that if we just believe enough we surely will beat the cancer. No. What we mean by this is that even in "loss," in Christ Jesus we have the victory. As the apostle Paul wrote to the Corinthians,

> For the trumpet will sound, and the dead will be raised imperishable, and we will be changed. For this perishable body must put on imperishability, and this mortal body must put on immortality.
>
> When this perishable body puts on imperishability, and this mortal body puts on immortality, then the saying that is written will be fulfilled:
> "Death has been swallowed up in victory."
> "Where, O death, is your victory?

Where, O death, is your sting?"
The sting of death is sin, and the power of sin is the law.
But thanks be to God, who gives us the victory through our
Lord Jesus Christ. (1 Cor. 15:52–57)

It is no surprise that this passage from 1 Corinthians is so often read at funerals, or at the graveside. This is the promise that accompanies us into and through the darkest valleys.

———

Karl has a very dear, old friend who fancies himself a real Bible believer, and Bible knower. He knows it better than you do—just ask him. This friend offered to pray over Karl (which Karl gladly accepted, even though it was, due to COVID and distance, a prayer prayed over the phone), and then encouraged him to trust God, believe in Jesus, and he would surely be alright. Karl, because he's just this kind of friend, responded by saying, "Don't worry, this illness does not lead to death." Karl's friend replied with a hearty, "Amen!" Karl then hung up the phone and had a little laugh to himself. Why? If you know the story of Jesus, Mary and Martha, and their brother Lazarus, you'll get it (if you don't know that story you can read it in the Gospel of John, chapter 11). What Karl was doing was quoting Jesus, who said, "This illness does not lead to death," about Lazarus. Lazarus, whose illness did in fact lead to death. But, because of the promises of God, made good through Jesus, death was not the end for Lazarus. Karl was leaning into that promise, that death is not the end for us. Because, to quote Paul again, "if we have been united with him in a death like his, we will certainly be united with him in a resurrection like his" (Rom. 6:5). Leaning into that

115

promise, a promise spoken into the uncertainty of the future and in the face of life's darkest valleys, is life giving, strengthening, calming. It makes it possible, and perhaps a bit easier, to go on living while you can.

––––––

MIKE (2022)

> O Lord, open my lips,
>     and my mouth will declare your praise. (Ps. 51:15)

The scriptural context of this text doesn't exactly match having cancer. The superscription designates Psalm 51 as part of David's confession of sin: "when the prophet Nathan came to him, after he had gone in to Bathsheba." Having come clean with the Lord and knowing God's steadfast faithfulness, David now asks God for redemption and renewal. David's words are part of a larger story. It is a story in which David has committed adultery with Bathsheba, who was already married to another man. Then, when Bathsheba becomes pregnant and David can't cover up the adultery, David arranges to have the other man, Uriah, killed in battle. The child that David and Bathsheba have then dies. David's suffering includes major league sin and major league suffering. But that's where these words "work" for me: In the face of suffering I found purpose, if not in the suffering itself, at least in my response to that suffering.

During my third of six chemo cycles at the St. Cloud Hospital, at zero dark thirty in the morning, I was reminded of an observation I had back during cycle 2. All my chemo had to be delivered in-patient, so every three weeks I got to spend Monday through Friday hospitalized, taking a five-day chemotherapy cocktail before I could go home. All of that was interspersed with massive doses of prednisone steroids to strengthen my body against the cancer as well as the hopeful cure. My bartenders were quick to keep my glass full, even without a tip on my part!

Fifth Floor North is the oncology ward at St. Cloud, so of course the place is crawling with IV stands and their attached computerized pump units. When something's not right, these pumps have a three-note alert tone, from low to high—which, I noticed, just so happens to be the first three notes for Morning Prayer, a traditional devotional prayer from the old green hymnal of my youth: "O, Lord, open my lips . . ."[1]

When my two older daughters, Laura and Anna, were up to hang out during their spring break, I pointed out the notes: "Sound familiar?" I asked. Both said yes but weren't sure why. I then sang, "O, Lord, open my lips . . . ," and they responded, "And my mouth shall declare your praise!" The notes were the same as those from the Morning Prayer liturgy that is used at a summer camp called Christikon—where both of them had worked and where our family often goes.

Later that day—we were still under COVID restrictions at the hospital and could have only two visitors at any given time—my youngest daughter, Eleanor, was there to repeat that call and response. She noted, as well, that those three notes are also the first notes to the Kyrie setting being used at the time at Trinity-Princeton in Sunday worship: "In peace let us pray to the Lord: Lord [*Kyrie*], have mercy."

How odd, yet wonderful, is that? The technical, medical necessity of an IV alert tone became for me the liturgical call to open my lips, so that my mouth might declare God's praise! It became the tritone call to pray to the Lord in peace. What occurred to me with those unexpected three notes, in this place and situation of suffering I'd rather not have been, is that the power, the grace, and the promised presence of the resurrected Christ came once again to me. The IV sounded the invitation to reconnect to the ritual and pattern of prayer. *And that ritual and pattern is part of what surprised and sustained me there.*

But in the midst of all the challenges of cancer, those three notes from a most unexpected source reminded me of my Lord's presence and called me back to the primary God-given reason for my life and, yes, even someday my death, wherever all this goes and however it ends: "O Lord, open my lips, and my mouth shall declare your praise. Glory to the Father, and to the Son, and to the Holy Spirit; as it was in the beginning, is now, and will be forever. Amen"—and even in spite of the timing of my initial treatments, the season of Lent—"Alleluia! Alleluia!"[2] Since then, Morning Prayer had become my own nearly daily discipline. Little did I know how important that refrain from Psalm 51 and Morning Prayer would become.

As I mentioned above, my family learned those notes at the summer camp called Christikon. There is a sign hanging over the front gate of that camp that isn't seen until you *leave* the camp, as one is *sent out*, whether that's on a backpacking trail or on the trail back home into the regular world: "Wherever you go Christ will go with you," the sign promises. O Lord, open my lips, and my mouth shall declare your praise.

Psalm 144 is another song of David, the warrior king:

> Blessed be the LORD, my rock,
> who trains my hands for war, and my fingers
> for battle;

> my rock and my fortress,
>   my stronghold and my deliverer,
> my shield, in whom I take refuge,
>   who subdues the peoples under me. (Ps. 144:1–2)

This being a psalm of David, the warrior and eventual king, I am certain that David's original intent for having hands trained for war and fingers ready for battle so that the peoples would be subdued under him is to be taken at face value.

My battle was not with people but with whatever was going on inside my body. There were countless nights of frustration and weariness and occasional pain and discomfort that had me crying like a little child. Writing, especially on my CaringBridge site, became therapeutic for me. And each one of my entries was "signed off" with this refrain from Psalm 144:1–2, less as a matter of bravado (which was often lacking) and more as a reminder, a hope, and a prayer.

---

## KARL (2022)

One of my greatest frustrations during my hospitalizations was that I couldn't read. I tried, but it was just too hard, first, because my vision was affected by the chemotherapy (Believe it or not, posttreatment, my vision is actually better—I am, as my optometrist put it, "Not insignificantly less nearsighted." How's that for a positive triple-negative?), and second, because I found it almost impossible to concentrate for any length of time. As a result, I didn't do a lot of Bible reading when I was in the hospital. But that doesn't mean that I was without God's Word. I turned, time and again, to the passages that I had memorized, and to the stories that were so familiar I could retell them almost word for word.

Two pieces in particular came to my mind often. The first was Daniel 3, the story of Shadrach, Meshach, and Abednego. Whether in the pages of the Bible itself, from memory, or (believe it or not) triggered by the Louis Armstrong song "Shadrach," or "Survival" by Bob Marley, or even the track from the Beastie Boys' album *Paul's Boutique*, this story has meant more to me than pretty much any other in the Bible.

The key element of the story lies between the theological question, asked arrogantly, contemptuously, by Nebuchadnezzar, and the response that Shadrach, Meshach, and Abednego make to the king. Lording his power over the three men, Nebuchadnezzar asks, "Who is the god that will deliver you out of my hands?" (Dan. 3:15). Shadrach, Meshach, and Abednego reply, "O Nebuchadnezzar, we have no need to present a defense to you in this matter. If our God whom we serve is able to deliver us from the furnace of blazing fire and out of your hand, O king, let him deliver us. But if not, be it known to you, O king, that we will not serve your gods and we will not worship the golden statue that you have set up" (3:16–18). In the face of cancer and uncertainty and abject powerlessness, this story has been so important to me because of this faith, shared by these three men. The faith of Shadrach, Meshach, and Abednego is the faith that I have wanted . . . needed. And, by the grace of God, it has been mine too, sustaining me and giving me strength.

Notice what the faith of Shadrach, Meshach, and Abednego looks like. They say very plainly, "if," and then, "if not." "If our God whom we serve is able to deliver us" out of the fire, and out of Nebuchadnezzar's power, well and good. "If . . ."

And they continue, "But if not," it makes no difference; our faith remains the Lord's. This is not some sort of transactional relationship, where the faith of Shadrach, Meshach, and Abednego is dependent on what God will do for them. This relationship is not based on some kind of quid pro quo. What they say is not "If . . . , then . . ."; rather it is, "If . . . , but if . . ." One way or the other, the relationship remains intact, the same.

Their faith is defined by trust, release, and peace. Trust: not presumption that something will be ours, but trust that come what may, God is with us. Release: freedom from the self-delusion that we will need to—let alone can—always have control. Peace: because of who God is, not what we do. This is faith at its deepest, and purest. And what this picture of faith is showing us is that this faith can be ours too.

How? How did Shadrach, Meshach, and Abednego find this sort of faith, and how can we? To be absolutely clear, I'm not saying that the faith of Shadrach, Meshach, and Abednego is a sort of model for what we need to be about, some kind of road map that we should follow, a behavior we need to emulate or an attitude we need to adopt. Rather, this faith is a gift that is ours for the having because of who God is and what God does. The secret to this faith lies in the background of the story. The key to this story lies not so much in fiery furnaces or angelic figures or mad kings, but in names.

The names Shadrach, Meshach, and Abednego are Babylonian names, and our three young men are not Babylonian but Jewish. Their original names, their true names, were taken from them by Nebuchadnezzar, changed when he gave them positions within his government. But though their names have been changed, their true names still define who they are at their core. Their true names are a testimony to their God. Shadrach's name is really Hananiah, which in Aramaic means "The Lord is gracious." Meshach's name is Mishael, which is a question asking, "Who is like God?" And Abednego's name is Azariah, "The Lord helps." Their names are confessions of faith, testimony to God as the source of their faithfulness. Or, perhaps better said, God's faithfulness makes their faithfulness possible. The deep, pure faith of Shadrach, Meshach, and Abednego is based not on their decision, or their attitude, or their effort, but on their God, a God who is gracious and incomparable, and who holds us close. Always.

And here is the most remarkable element of the whole story: Shadrach, Meshach, and Abednego believe that no matter what happens, come what may, God is trustworthy, faithful in all things, even, it seems, when it comes to death. Even when we face death, our gracious, incomparable God holds us close. As our teacher Dick Nysse said of this story, "Death does not limit or end God's capacity to create a future."[3] This is who God is and what God does—wringing life out of death, forgiving sin, banishing fear, raising to new life. This is who God is and what God does. And if we know this God, the God of life, the God who stops at nothing to reach us, the God who loves raising people from the dead, then we, too, can know this faith. It is ours for the having.

One last word is key for me. It does not come directly from the story, but as a believer in Jesus, for me it is the inevitable conclusion. King Nebuchadnezzar, in his presumption and arrogance, in the deluded claim that the power is his, asks, "Who is the god that will deliver you?" And we have the ultimate answer: Jesus, who gave sight to the blind, the power to walk to the lame, and hearing to the deaf. Jesus, who gives his body and blood for us sinners. Jesus, who said, "If it is possible, let this cup pass from me," but if not . . . (Matt. 26:39). Jesus, whose name in Hebrew is *Yeshua*, which means "He will save." Who is the God who will save you? We know this God. He is Christ Jesus; he will save.

The other piece of Scripture that I turned to regularly was Psalm 118. Psalm 118 is a liturgy of thanksgiving; it is also one of the messianic psalms—psalms that anticipate and celebrate the promised messiah. If Psalm 110:1 is the Old Testament verse most often quoted in the New Testament, then Psalm 118 has what are probably two of the most recognizable, most familiar passages quoted in the New Testament. They go like this:

> The stone that the builders rejected
>> has become the chief cornerstone.
> This is the LORD's doing;
>> it is marvelous in our eyes. (Ps. 118:22–23)

And,

> Save us, we beseech you, O LORD!
>> O LORD, we beseech you, give us success!
> Blessed is the one who comes in the name
>> of the LORD.
>> We bless you from the house of the LORD.
>> (Ps. 118:25–26)

If we follow the Gospel of Mark, these two quotations come to us in reverse order. Verses 25–26 are sung to Jesus as he makes his way into Jerusalem in Mark 11, and they sound like this:

> [Jesus and the disciples] were approaching Jerusalem. . . . Many people spread their cloaks on the road, and others spread leafy branches that they had cut in the fields. Then those who went ahead and those who followed were shouting,
>> "Hosanna!
>>> Blessed is the one who comes in the name of the Lord!
>>> Blessed is the coming kingdom of our ancestor David!
>> Hosanna in the highest heaven!" (Mark 11:1, 7–10)

The quotation here of Psalm 118 may sound a little different, but it is actually much closer than it seems. Psalm 118:25 says, "Save us, we beseech you," which comes to us in Mark 11:9 from the Hebrew of the Old Testament, by way of New Testament Greek, as "Hosanna!" But "Hosanna" is not so much a translation as it is a transliteration—where a word comes to us from another language and isn't translated, it's simply adopted, and its meaning is brought over. Words like "karaoke," "angst," "café," "bazaar," "plaza"—words that have a certain . . . je ne sais quoi. In the case of "Hosanna" we have such a loanword, which comes all the way to English by way of Greek: the Hebrew הוֹשִׁיעָה נָּא (hoshi'ah na') becomes Ὡσαννά (Hōsanna), which becomes "Hosanna." "Hosanna," transliterated and sung, is heard as a shout of joy; "Hosanna" translated means, "Save us, we beseech you!" This quotation is a cry of both joy and entreaty, and it is taken up in all four of the Gospels. This is how—these are the words with which—the people greeted Jesus as he rode into Jerusalem.

These familiar verses from Psalm 118:25–26 are sung about Jesus, and to Jesus. And this dialectic that "Hosanna" expresses, both joy and a plea for help, fits perfectly with what Jesus teaches about who he is. Three times in the Gospel of Mark Jesus talks about what he has come to endure:

> He began to teach them that the Son of Man must undergo great suffering, and be rejected by the elders, the chief priests, and the scribes, and be killed, and after three days rise again. He said all this quite openly. (Mark 8:31–32)

> The Son of Man is to be betrayed into human hands, and they will kill him, and three days after being killed, he will rise again. (Mark 9:31)

> See, we are going up to Jerusalem, and the Son of Man will be handed over to the chief priests and the scribes, and they will condemn him to death; then they will hand him over to the Gentiles; they will mock him, and spit upon him, and flog him, and kill him; and after three days he will rise again. (Mark 10:33–34)

Jesus tells us that the victory he brings, the success he offers, goes first through the valley of the shadow of death, first to rejection and suffering, first to the cross and death, first to the grave. Only then to victory. And this is why, in the throes of my darkest days, these verses from Psalm 118 rang in my mind and heart as true: joy in the promise, and the plea for that promise to be fulfilled.

And in the midst of it all, the verse from Psalm 118 that gets skipped as it is sung by crowds in Mark stood out for me—in a spirit not unlike the faith of Shadrach, Meshach, and Abednego—as the way to entrust things to God's faithfulness.

Psalm 118:24 goes like this,

> This is the day that the LORD has made;
>     let us rejoice and be glad in it.

"This is the day that the LORD has made"; *this* is the day—today, not just that day way back when, not just a day in some future, this is the day. *This* is the day, whatever the day might bring.

---

## ROLF (1986)

I was just shy of my seventeenth birthday when they amputated my second leg in 1982. And I was just past my eighteenth birthday, in 1983, when I had the last of my teenage lung surgeries. I think that this was the twelfth lung surgery I had endured, so I was used to the surgeries by then. After each of the first two lung surgeries in 1981, it took me two weeks to recover. But by 1983, I had the recovery process down and could be back in school or back at work after just a week. On August 1, 1983, my dad had a sabbatical starting at the University of St. Andrews in Scotland. (The fact that St. Andrews is also the birthplace of golf and that my dad was once pretty near a scratch golfer had nothing to do with it, I'm sure.) I arranged my summer to have the surgery the last week of July, because there were other things I wanted to do. So my parents agreed on the timing. I went through surgery and got out to the intensive care unit for recovery. My parents saw that I made it through surgery, kissed me on the forehead, and headed to the airport.

Some friends and other folk said to my parents, "You can't take your sabbatical now! Rolf's in the hospital!" Others said, "Rolf is leaving for college next month. How is he going to move into the dorm? By himself!?"

My mom said, "He'll be fine. The timing was his choice. And he knows how to do this by now. He'll figure it out." So they boarded a jet plane and headed to the land of heather, golf, and whiskey. After I went through a week of recovery, my friend Laura brought me home from the hospital. I then ignored doctor's orders not to drive for two weeks. And when it was time to leave for college, Gene and Sharon Jasnoch, my dear friend Jay's parents, drove me to college and helped me move into the concrete bunker known as Brady Hall.

I love that my parents trusted me enough to let me make my own choices, to figure out how to live my life in a wheelchair without hovering over me, and to make whatever arrangements I needed to make. I didn't always make wise decisions, but that's part of life too. A few years later I went to Germany by myself. Again, people said to my mom, "Really!? You're letting Rolf go to Germany alone?" "I'm not letting him go, it's his choice," she said. "But I approve. He can do it."

During those years of almost constant surgery and chemotherapy—two amputations, three separate courses of chemo, ten random-but-related surgeries, and twelve lung resections—my official chance of survival was "lower than a snake's belly in a wagon rut." That's not official Mayo Clinic terminology, but it's what my future father-in-law would have said.

I went to college in St. Paul, Minnesota, which at the time was about a two-hour drive from the Mayo Clinic. During my first year, I would drive to Mayo one day every couple of months for my checkups—blood work, X-ray, CT scan of the abdomen (which at the time took forty-five to sixty minutes while contorted in a painful position), and physical exam. By sophomore year, because the checkups were clear, they came every three months. By junior year, they were every four months.

After my junior year, in July of 1986—three years after that last lung surgery—I had a checkup. Again, it was clear. The doctors told me based on statistics—three years of clear checkups since the last metastasis—that it was very likely that I was cured of my cancer. The war with cancer was over—and even though I had lost every battle to cancer, somehow I had won the war.

That night was peak Minnesota weather. It was warm but not hot, with a clear sky and gentle breeze. I was sitting in the lower quad of my college campus with my friend Julie. I told her my good news, and she said, "No excuses now."

"No excuses now." Those were wonderful words. In just three words she was saying, "Your cancer is behind you. You now have a future beyond cancer to live for, to prepare for, to plan for, and to face head-on. It's time to get after it."

The worst part of my life was over, but in some ways, the hardest part was about to begin. I had one year of college left, and then what? When my wife, daughter, and I dropped my son off for college, he said to our daughter (she later told us), "So I guess my childhood is over." Well, maybe for some,

128

college is the start of adult life. It wasn't for me. For me, it was a four-year extension of young adult life—I wasn't a child anymore, but I wasn't an adult either. With one year left of college and a clean bill of health, I now knew that the future I had been hoping would happen was now a reality.

And here's the thing. For the first time since I had been diagnosed with cancer, I was *existentially afraid*. While I had cancer, I was often afraid of certain procedures I had to face—such as the "red death" chemo, the pain of the next lung surgery, or certain invasive procedures of which I will spare you the details. But I was never existentially afraid of dying. I even once told my mother, "I know that one day I am going to die. But *I am not going to die of cancer!*" It made her cry. But years later, when I was declared in the clear, she reminded me of that conversation. I had not forgotten, either.

But suddenly, I was afraid. I was afraid of what a long-term life with no legs in a wheelchair would be like. Would I find a wife? (Side note: It was *really* hard trying to figure out how to date as a guy with no legs.) Would I find a job that I could do and also enjoy? Would I find a place to live? I decided to go to seminary—but would a church ever hire a guy with no legs? I had never seen a church that didn't have at least three steps up to the chancel (that's fancy church crazy talk for the front of the church) and even more steps up to the altar and pulpit (that's even more fancy church crazy talk for the table and the podium).[4] I simply did not know what would become of me. For the first time I was *existentially afraid*. I wasn't afraid of dying. *I was afraid of living!*

In those next three to four years, as I lived with this new existential fear of living, one Bible passage really spoke to me and gave me courage and hope. It wasn't Jeremiah 29:11 (look it up); it was Psalm 27:1–4.

> The LORD is my light and my salvation;
>    whom shall I fear?
> The LORD is the stronghold of my life;
>    of whom shall I be afraid?
> When evildoers assail me
>    to devour my flesh—
> my adversaries and foes—
>    they shall stumble and fall.
> Though an army encamp against me,
>    my heart shall not fear;
> though war rise up against me,
>    yet I will be confident.
> One thing I asked of the LORD,
>    that will I seek after:
> to live in the house of the LORD
>    all the days of my life,
> to behold the beauty of the LORD,
>    and to inquire in his temple.

These verses spoke to me and for me. I prayed the psalm and leaned into it. It told the truth about life and God twice. It said that there are things in life that are worth fearing: armies (literal or figurative) that encamp against us, adversaries and foes (physical, spiritual, metaphorical) that we must face, wars (like cancer) that rise up against us. But because the Lord is with us—because the Lord is our light, our salvation, our stronghold—we need not fear. Yes, there are things worth fearing, *but we need not live in fear*, because the Lord is with us. We can be confident as we face life because the Lord is with us.

And one more thing. There is beauty. There is beauty in the world, in life, and there is beauty for you. Even if most of the world might think a person who is disfigured by disability and illness is ugly, with the Lord there is beauty. "One thing I asked of the LORD, that I will seek after: to live in the house of the LORD all the days of my life, to behold the beauty of the LORD" (Ps. 27:4). Even though one cannot see the Lord, the Lord is beautiful. And with the Lord in one's life, there is a beauty that overshadows all the shadows we might fear. A friend and fellow band member of mine named Steve Thompson wrote a song about becoming spiritually aware of the beauty that is all around us. The song is called "The Light of Love Comes Shining Through." Here are the bridge and final chorus of the song about a vision he perceived of being surrounded by a glorious ocean of color-transcending, divine beauty:

> Luminous ocean—nature's spectrum transcending;
> Waves of heaven's light break over time and space;
> 'Til faithful eyes through tears see it unending;
> Baptizing all creation in a lustrous flood of grace.
>
> There is glory all around,
> Ever bright and pure and true!
> All the barriers will come down.
> As the light of love comes shining through,
> The light of love comes shining through![5]

# 6

# Death

Recurrence, Fear, Exhaustion, and Hope

Come to me, all you who are weary and are carrying heavy burdens, and I will give you rest. Take my yoke upon you, and learn from me, for I am gentle and humble in heart, and you will find rest for your souls. For my yoke is easy, and my burden is light.

—Matthew 11:28–30 NRSVue

Who will separate us from the love of Christ? Will hardship, or distress, or persecution, or famine, or nakedness, or peril, or sword? . . . For I am convinced that neither death, nor life, nor angels, nor rulers, nor things present, nor things to come, nor powers, nor height, nor depth, nor anything else in all creation, will be able to separate us from the love of God in Christ Jesus our Lord.

—Romans 8:35, 38–39

133

## ROLF (2007)

In June 2007, I was looking forward to a weekend family vacation in central Minnesota, which was to be followed by a weeklong working trip to Indiana with my friend Andy (whose wife was "way pregnant," as we say in Minnesota). My seasonal allergies were nagging; I had a persistent cough. A student, Marc, dropped by my office to talk. I said, "Can we sit outside in the sun? It's a little chilly in here."

Marc looked stunned. "You're cold? It's not chilly in here. And it's 90 degrees outside. You should go see a doctor."

My wife was due to return that evening from a business trip, so my brother Karl and sister Karen watched my kids while I went to the only urgent care I could find open. The X-ray showed a shadow in my right lung, so the doctor told me to see my primary care doctor as soon as possible. "I'm looking forward to a trip to Indiana next week," I said. "Can this wait?" He looked at me carefully and said very slowly, "I wouldn't leave town."

The next day was a Friday. My primary care doctor fit me in and scheduled a CT scan for Monday—the day before my trip to Indiana. My wife, Amy, and our kids, Ingrid (eight) and Gunnar (three), took our weekend trip. Amy and the kids planned to stay at the resort for the full week along with her parents, while I went to Indiana.

On Monday, I had the CT scan and then drove to see my doc. She said, "This is never easy. The CT shows a very large tumor in your right lung."

It was a beautiful, blue, summer day. And out of that blue summer sky came some cold, stormy, November news. I was shocked.

I was forty-two years old. And twenty-seven years after my original diagnosis—and twenty-one years since I had been told I was out of the woods—my childhood cancer was back.

I had been living mostly without fear of cancer for over twenty years. Once you've had cancer, you never really live without fear of it. Even after years, a slightly swelling mass in your neck or abdomen can send you scurrying to the doctors. But I had not been thinking daily about cancer for many years.

And now it was back. So was the fear. But the fear was a bigger, hairier, uglier fear than the adolescent fear I'd shrugged off two decades earlier. This was an adult fear—because I now had a wife and two young children to care for.

I got in the car for the five-minute drive home and called my wife. Through tears, I told her the news. Then I called my friend Andy to tell him he would have to make the trip on his own. When he answered the phone, his first words were: "I've got bad news." Correctly guessing that his wife's water had broken and he couldn't make the trip, I said, "I've got worse." The doctor was right. I wasn't leaving town.

I called my mom and dad, who said they'd be right over.

No sooner had I reached home than my friend Hans called and said, "I'm coming over."

I said, "Why?"—because I incorrectly guessed Amy wouldn't have had time to call him.

"Because you're screwed up," he said through tears. *Because you're screwed up.* Those were some of the most loving words a friend has ever said to me.

My wife moved fast. She called my work, and my friend Diane brought dinner. Amy and the kids were home within four hours.

Mayo Clinic can move fast. I was assigned one of the best surgeons. They scheduled a thoracotomy (my twelfth or thirteenth—I'd honestly lost track after ten) for that Friday. The surgeon informed me that the cough I'd been enduring wasn't due to allergies but was caused by the tumor, which had invaded my diaphragm. The chill I had was actually a pretty robust fever—my body trying to fight what was actually a very large tumor. The surgeon explained that the tumor might be wrapped about my inferior vena cava—the largest vein in one's body, which carries oxygen-depleted blood back to the heart. If that was the case, he said, they were going to have to do some tricky reconstructive work, and there was a risk of death.

The day before the surgery, I played with my kids and wrote them a letter, which I sealed and gave to my wife. Since you're reading this, you know that I didn't die. The surgery went even better than could have been hoped. My kids never had to open the letter. I think my wife still has it tucked away somewhere.

The surgeon sent me to see a new oncologist. One whom he described as knowing more about sarcoma than anyone else in the world. His wife calls him Scott. I called him Dr. Sarcoma.

Dr. Sarcoma informed me that the tumor in my right lung had been there and growing for twenty-seven years. For a good twenty-six years, it was so microscopically small that it could not be detected by CT scan. And then it started to grow faster. "Why," I asked, "did it start to grow faster?"

"We don't know," he said. "But there's a pretty good chance that there was only one tumor left." He then offered to mix me a cocktail of chemotherapy drugs—he probably had the red devil, the white Cytoxan, and other fun chemicals from my past in mind.

"I'm good," I said. "I prefer to mix my own cocktails made of over-the-counter chemicals. I use a lot of lime."

He also informed me that I was a world-record holder. I held the record for the longest lapse between initial diagnosis and a late sarcoma metastasis. This tumor was 26.5 years after my initial diagnosis and almost 24 years since my last lung tumor was resected. He mentioned that some poser in Germany had gone about 18 years between diagnosis and late-life recurrence. My 24- and 26-year gap blew him out of the water. (Okay, Dr. Sarcoma didn't say it with quite that eloquence.)

So I am a world-record holder. It's a record nobody wants. There is no gold medal, no podium, and no Wikipedia page. But still, being alive to claim the "longest" record sure beats the alternative. Thanks be to God.

There's a great deal more I could write about 2007 (such as the seminary colleague who drove to Mayo Clinic to preach me a sermon while I was still on morphine; I kept nodding off and my wife kept laughing—he preached on Psalm 104). But this is enough.

The *shock*. The *out-of-nowhere return* of the old enemy. The new, *adult* level of fear. Those are some of the main headlines.

———

Fear can play an important and positive role in our lives. Fear can be really good for us. Some theorists posit that fear is an emotion or mental state that has been refined through evolution. When some stimulus or situation triggers fear, it can either save us from a dangerous situation or help minimize the harm we might experience. The emotion of fear can steer us away from *doing something dangerous* (like licking a frozen fire hydrant), from *going somewhere dangerous* (like walking into a Chicago Bears bar while wearing a Minnesota Vikings jersey), or from certain *interactions with dangerous people* (like a chainsaw battle with a guy with a hockey goalie mask, or going in with a Sicilian when death is on the line).

In the early years after Rolf developed bone cancer, every time Karl, who was five years younger, felt the slightest twinge of bone pain, their mom rushed Karl in to see the doctor. It was a bit of an overreaction. But it was an overreaction caused by fear. It's only paranoia if they really aren't out to get you. And it's only hypochondria if you really aren't sick.

During those same years, fear was Rolf's invisible friend. Like most invisible friends, it wasn't always there. Or maybe it is better to say that the fear wasn't always palpable, although it was always there—humming lowly in the background, like an air conditioner on a hot summer day. But the fear was there. And then, at certain times, the fear would pop up. Some occasions became predictable—such as the regular checkups at Mayo.

From November 1980 through July 1986, Rolf's life was measured by the regular, routine checkups at Mayo. It became a ritual of sorts. Rise early, before the sun. Drive down highway 52 and park. Check in for bloodwork, CT scan, and X-ray. Breakfast at the Kahler Grand Hotel's first-floor cafe. Find a way to kill six or seven hours without spending (much) money. See the oncologist. And, if necessary (which it often was), see the surgeon. Drive home.

If there was good news—"No sign of cancer"—Rolf would experience an almost audible release of tension in his body.

He would then realize that over the past week or so, the stress had been building up. The fear. And if there was bad news— "We see nodules on both lungs"—the fear would slap Rolf on the back and say, "Ha! Thought you were rid of me? Not hardly!"

In chapter 2, Mike recalled how at night, his mind would race and he couldn't sleep. The "what-ifs"—the fear—would dominate his thinking. He told his father-in-law, who was also a cancer survivor, "I couldn't get my brain to turn off and let go of all the 'what-ifs'!" His father-in-law responded, "That never really goes away." In other words, the fear never really goes away.

The Bible has a couple of deep truths to teach about fear.

The first deep truth about fear comes from Proverbs and is a bit abstract. Maybe even a bit confusing. The book of Proverbs says this in two similar ways: "The fear of the LORD is the beginning of knowledge" (1:7a). "The fear of the LORD is the beginning of wisdom" (9:10a). In the Hebrew of the Old Testament, the word translated here as "fear" can mean regular old "fear," but it can also mean "awe," "reverence," or "respect." So this is often translated as "Reverence for the LORD is the beginning of wisdom."

From a spiritual perspective, the deep truth is that *no matter how big your fears are, there is One who is bigger than all your fears: the Lord.* And with the Lord in your life, you can learn to give all of your fears away. If life gives you fear, give that fear to God. Sort of like regifting the ugly sweater you received last Christmas, you can regift your fear to God. Knowing that there is a living God who is bigger than your fears can allow a person to live daily life in the shadow of fear without letting fear overshadow daily life.

The second deep truth about fear comes from the Psalms and is less abstract. More specifically, it comes from the psalms of trust. The psalms of trust paradoxically *name the terrifying realities all around us* and, at the same time, name the presence of the Lord as a reason not to fear. The lesson here is that being honest about our fears is the first step in facing those fears . . . and facing them down. The psalms of trust do not deny fears. They do the exact opposite! The psalms of trust name the fears. Consider these lines from well-known trust psalms:

> Even though I walk through the darkest valley,
>   I fear no evil,
> for you are with me. (Ps. 23:4a)

> Though an army encamp against me,
>   my heart will not fear;
> though war rise up against me,
>   Even then, I will trust. (Ps. 27:3; our translation)

> God is our refuge and strength,
>   a clear help, found in troubles.
> Therefore, we do not fear when the earth quakes,
>   when mountains shake in the heart of the seas,
> when its waters rage and roil,
>   when mountains heave with its arrogance!
>     (Ps. 46:1–3; our translation)

Notice how the psalm writers do not deny, ignore, minimize, or deflect away from the things that terrify them. No! Quite the opposite! They name their fears. They describe them carefully—drawing upon rich, poetic description: "When mountains shake in the heart of the seas, when its waters rage and roil, when mountains heave with its arrogance!" The lesson is clear: Face your fears. Name them. Do not deny, deflect, or diminish them. Look them in the figurative eye. Maybe even spit at them. (Not literally—that would be gross.)

How can you do that? How can you spit in cancer's eye? You can do so because the Lord is on your side—"a clear help, found in troubles," as Psalm 46 puts it. In the New Testament, St. Paul basically writes his own version of a psalm of trust in Philippians 4. He is writing *from prison*. He acknowledges knowing what it is to *be in need*, to *have little*, to *go hungry*, and to *be in distress*. In the middle of acknowledging all of these fearful realities, Paul writes—in a verse that is basically always taken out of context—"I can do all things through him who strengthens me" (Phil. 4:13). Paul was not bragging that he was Superman—that he could literally do anything. Rather, Paul was expressing his trust in God. That through Jesus Christ, who strengthens him, he could face any of the fearful realities that he would have to face: hunger, having little, being imprisoned, perhaps even being placed on trial with life and death hanging in the balance.

With confidence that God is present, we can face our fears head-on.

---

## KARL (VIA ROLF) (2024)

Note to the reader: Throughout this book, we have had first-name headings—Rolf, Mike, Karl—at the start of sections in which each of us then tells our story in the first person. For reasons that will be made clear later in this chapter, Rolf needed to write some parts of Karl's story in this chapter in the third person.

Early in 2024, Karl began working toward returning to full-time ministry. But from the perspective of his health, the buildup didn't go as well as he had hoped. He just didn't have the physical and emotional strength to serve as lead pastor in ways that the congregation needed or that he could take pride in. After family dinner on one Thursday evening in Lent, Angela asked Karl, "Where are you right now?" Karl looked up and realized that he couldn't recall what they had just eaten for dinner. After discerning with Angela, he realized that he needed to step down from his call as lead pastor. In his letter of resignation to the congregation, Karl included these words:

> This decision, which I have not come to lightly, is, I believe, in the best interest of the congregation, and of myself, my wife Angela, and our family.
>
> Since my return from illness just over a year ago I have been working to build my strength and stamina, and to increase my time at work. This has been a slow, if steady, process for the most part, and had been promising. At the beginning of this calendar year, I began to intentionally increase my time, arriving at essentially full-time towards the end of Lent and Holy Week. It had been my hope to return to full-time ministry with the arrival of Easter. As Holy Week approached, however, it became clear to me that I had hit a wall in my capacity, and found that I was increasingly fatigued. My conclusion is that, as of now, I simply do not have what it takes to fulfill the responsibilities of this call. Good Shepherd deserves more, and so does my family.

I am grateful for my colleagues on staff, and for our congregation's leadership for their patience as I have been recovering and working my way back. I have taken that opportunity seriously, and am deeply, deeply appreciative.

Looking back on the past eleven years, I must say that I am grateful as well for the time we have shared together. Thank you for your support not only in these past two years as I have dealt with leukemia, but for the ways in which we have lived and worked together for the gospel. This congregation has been a wonderful call for me, a refuge in many ways for my children, and a place—a people—where I clearly see a faith that works.

As of now, I do not know what will be next for me. I know that I am not done in terms of my work in the church, but as to what is next, we will have to wait and see. Whatever is next, for me and for Good Shepherd, is safely in God's hands.

The day that Karl announced he needed to resign as senior pastor at the Lutheran Church of the Good Shepherd in May 2024, he got a call from Pastor Dave Lose from Mount Olivet Lutheran Church. Would Karl be interested in joining the pastoral team at Mount Olivet, perhaps in a part-time role? After some discernment work, Karl said yes. He would need to take the summer off to recover his strength, but then he could start part-time in September.

Karl endeavored to spend most of the summer at our father's lake place on Mule Lake, Minnesota—reading, resting, and starting to write this book.

Karl's last Sunday at Good Shepherd was May 19, 2024—Pentecost Sunday. As you can imagine, the turnout was large, and the sanctuary was full. At one point in the service, Karl joked, "It's such a great turnout, I'm going to quit again next week." His sermon was marked, as usual, by his sense of humor and the clarity with which Karl spoke the promises of God. After playing a quick clip from fellow leukemia victim Steve Goodman's song "You Never Even Called Me by My Name," in which Goodman and John Prine tried to include every stereotypical element of a country song, Karl began his sermon:

In the Spirit of Steve Goodman and in this, my last sermon with you all, it's my last chance to say to you everything I've ever wanted to say. Eleven years' worth! Buckle up.

First, you belong to God.

The final picture of Karl as pastor at Good Shepherd was taken by his son, Sam. It shows Karl on the dock at Mule Lake, still fully robed as if for Sunday morning—white robe, green stole—but with a fishing hat on his head, a red-and-white bobber on his stole, and a fishing pole in his hand, ready to make a cast (see p. vii). The message was clear. Karl was taking a break from fishing for people, and for the summer at least, Karl would be fishing for fish.

A couple of weeks later, Karl got some great news from his oncologist. On June 14, 2024, Karl posted the following on his CaringBridge page:

Hobbits enjoy second breakfast. Bone marrow transplant-ees enjoy second birthdays. When we get new bone marrow, it's like a new birth, and so in some ways the odometer starts at zero again.

On June 12th, I went in for my annual bone marrow biopsy to test for any sign of leukemia, or of my genetic mutation, the Philadelphia+ chromosome. Two key test results are in, and positive. Which is to say, negative—no apparent sign of either.

And so, today marks my second second birthday. I don't remember my first second birthday, so I plan to make my second second birthday memorable. Totally two. TERRIBLE.

- Today I will have a tantrum, for no reason.
- Today I will fight nap time, tooth and claw, and then crash for a monster nap.
- Today I will demand Dairy Queen. For dinner.
- I will glory in my two-ness, with a childlike faith, and a grateful heart for good results. Thanks be to God, and great medical (and family and friend) care.

In other anniversary news, next week Angela and I will mark our 10th wedding anniversary. I am so glad to be here for it, and so glad to have her in my life.

Thank you, AFJ, for everything. I love you.

---

## MIKE (2024)

August 28, 2022, was my return to the parish. While I had hoped it would be along the lines of MacArthur's victorious return to the Philippines in World War II, it was anything but. For one, there were a whole host of swirling postpandemic issues for my congregation that in my absence were coming to a head. And, more personally, there were swirling questions in my heart and mind about what my return would even mean or look like. Yes, my lymphoma was in remission. Yes, I was free from the intensity of the chemo

145

treatments as well as the weekly regimen of meds intended
to help my body cope with the chemo. But one does not
simply walk into Mordor. One does not come through a
whole-life-impacting ordeal like that without being changed
in some way. Having spent the last six months, or certainly
the first three months of that term, fighting for my life,
could I care about the issues that a postpandemic ELCA
(Evangelical Lutheran Church in America) congregation
needed their pastor to care about? Would my remissioned-
but-diminished physical health allow me to return to any
sort of even a shadow of what I once knew as vibrant and
normal, addled as I was with the forgetfulness and brain fog
of the so-called "chemo brain" and saddled with the weekly
bouts of a fatigue that all the naps and all the coffee in the
world could not even dent? I had struggled before over the
previous decade or so with vocation. But those struggles
were mostly over and around, to borrow from The Clash,
"should I stay or should I go now" from the particular setting
where I was serving. This was something different: a general
fear about "What's next?" and specific fears about "Could I
even continue being a pastor?"; and, "If so, what would that
look like in my diminished capacity, especially in a setting
that needed an undiminished pastor?"; or worse yet, "If I
can't continue in parish ministry, what *could* I do?" I have
all the privileged, middle-class responsibilities and hopes
anyone else has—kids in college, a mortgage, retirement
hopes. Is this how ruin begins? The immediate fear (realized or not) of bumps and aches and pains and the thoughts
of "Is it back?"—a fear about which I now knew its medical
redress, the procedures, the characters, the tastes and smells
and more and wanted to avoid, well, like the plague—had

been swallowed up by a bigger fear with fewer answers or known steps.

And yet, even for you to read that paragraph is for you to be invited into "the answer" to that fear. Granted, it is not an "answer" that solves everything or makes the fear go away forever or ends with, "And they all lived happily ever after." Rather, what you are reading, both in whole and in the individual specifics of our stories, are the ways that three sinners who are followers of Jesus Christ have responded to our fears.

Two key spiritual perspectives have already been offered as fear's redress. The first was that no matter how big your fears are, there is One who is bigger than all your fears: the Lord; that with the Lord in your life, you can learn to give all of your fears away; and that knowing that there is a living God who is bigger than your fears can allow a person to live daily life in the shadow of fear. VeggieTales is *right*! "God *is* bigger than the Boogieman!" For nearly thirty years, I have staked my very living in proclaiming in a hundred different ways to any who would listen and hear that, because of the cross and resurrection of Christ, fear and death—the biggest fear of them all—are not the final words in our lives. Preaching this is one thing; believing it, living and dying it, is quite another.

The second deep spiritual truth about fear from the psalms of trust is to name the terrifying realities all around us and in so doing to name the presence of the Lord as a reason not to fear, or at least, to know and trust or even perhaps hope that the Lord and the Lord's presence are indeed bigger. Here is in some way the nuts and bolts of our ordeals and how Karl, Rolf, and I have named and given our fears to God: "Is it back?" "What's next?" "Could I even continue being a pastor?" "If so, what would that look like in my diminished capacity, especially in a setting that needs an undiminished pastor?" "If I can't continue in parish ministry, what *could* I do?" These have been just some of the names of our fears, and even in our suffering and our naming of those fears we have experienced the living Lord Jesus Christ, crucified and raised from the dead.

I can't necessarily give you a step-by-step process of what this looked like for me. In no small way, this book is part of that process of remembering the Lord's presence throughout our ordeals and naming those fears. The psalms themselves at times model that memory: "I remembered you, God, and I groaned; I meditated, and my spirit grew faint," Psalm 77:3 declares (NIV); "I remember the days of long ago; I meditate on all your works and consider what your hands have done," proclaims Psalm 143:5 (NIV).

But here is what that has looked like for me from my return to parish ministry to now: Each month in the congregation I was serving at the time, the council president and I would meet to set the agenda for our upcoming council meetings. As I continued to struggle physically and mentally and pastorally through my recovery, I took our council's president into confidence in the spring of 2023, probably about six months after my return. "I don't have any active plans to leave. But we all have to discern and recognize that I might not be the person who can serve this congregation in the way that it needs." Similarly, I began to pack my parachute by enrolling in a mostly online certification course that would equip me for potential intentional interim ministry.

Again, I had no active plans to leave. But I was also more acutely feeling the disconnect between the congregation's needs and my ability and will to respond, especially in my diminished capacity to be the pastor I was before cancer or even the pandemic. I was feeling increasingly worn and nearly burned out. As Bilbo Baggins reflected to Gandalf about the burden of having carried the One Ring for many years, "I feel all thin, sort of *stretched*, if you know what I mean: like butter scraped over too much bread."[1] Though it didn't carry me to where I thought I might be headed, the interim ministry coursework helped in my discernment process: If I couldn't handle normal parish ministry in my present condition, there was no way I would be any good in trying to serve congregations in need of intentional, often-crisis-management interim ministry. This became even more magnified as a new burden and a new set of fears began to rise as my father began to enter end-stage dementia after nearly a decade of failing health.

In January of 2024 a friend and ministry colleague of mine called me up. "I hear you've been considering interim ministry," she said and went on to say that she had a potential gig for me at the congregation she was serving as interim lead.

"Connie, I'm toeing the line of burnout right now," I told her. "And I don't know how wise it is"—this is an expression of fear—"for me to take another call where I might be burned out in a new, unfamiliar setting and relationship, when at least I and this congregation I'm serving now know and trust each other."

"Well, here's what we would want you to do," she replied. "We would want you to serve as a bridge pastor on an interim basis, simply to take your turn at preaching and leading worship; be a part of our general pastoral care and visitation; and coordinate our adult education."

Here was a call to the simplicity of parish ministry. And I would say that these are the top three things I love about parish ministry and that led me to parish ministry. They are also my top competencies.

"I'll at least sit for an interview," I told her.

To name the terrifying realities all around us and in so doing to name the presence of the Lord as a reason not to fear, or at least, to know and trust or even perhaps hope, can also be an act of confessional faith, that the Lord and the Lord's presence are indeed bigger.

On Sunday, April 14, 2024, I preached my last sermon at Trinity Lutheran Church.

On Saturday, April 20, I began an interim ministry at Zion Lutheran Church in Anoka, Minnesota.

As it turns out, I was a failure at temporary bridge pastoring: After nearly six months of interim ministry, on September 29, 2024, the Zion congregation voted to extend a permanent call to me as an associate pastor. God is good.

Here's the thing, though. While the immediate fears of my vocation, my recovery, and how those fit together may be relieved, the unknown—as it does for every human being—still remains. December of 2023 featured a biopsy of an enlarged lymph node in my groin area that my semiannual CT scan picked up. It wasn't enlarged enough to warrant any concern from my oncologist. But after what I've gone through, any enlargement is concerning for Kari and me. The biopsy came back negative, but my most recent scan indicated an additional slight enlargement, with my consult with my oncologist pending. To say this doesn't weigh on my psyche would be a lie. Likewise, while the time between my bouts with fatigue has lengthened and their duration shortened—which my oncologist says could eventually go away, or it could just be my new normal—they still occur, especially as I have continued to grow stronger out of recovery and find myself pushing to resume anything that feels like normal precancer activity. (Most days, cancer is far from my mind and has instead been replaced with other thoughts and realities.)

One of my first home visits after returning to the parish in 2022 was with an elderly parishioner named Margaret. Margaret knows her Bible backward and forward and has herself faced a lifetime of trials and fears. When I brought her the Lord's Supper and devotions in her home, Margaret presented me with a ceramic refrigerator magnet inscribed with Psalm 46:1, "God is our refuge and strength, a very present help in trouble," a verse I knew to have been Margaret's confirmation verse. "I know you know what this means," she said as I opened the box. That magnet still hangs in my office. It always will.

––––––

### KARL (VIA ROLF) (2024)

Karl had decided to spend as much time as he could in June and July at our dad's cabin on Mule Lake in Minnesota—resting, reading, writing, and fishing.

I was able to bust away from work and join Karl and Dad a bit in both June and July. Summer started off well, with Karl's positive oncology report and the call for him to join the staff at Mount Olivet. Karl and his wife, Angela, celebrated their tenth wedding anniversary at Sommer Ro, a 120-year-old cabin our great-grandparents had built in Wisconsin—which somehow still exists and is still in the (very extended) family. Karl and Angela had been married there in 2014. Karl and I were also looking forward to our annual week of study and fellowship in August with six pastor friends at Sommer Ro. Each year, we choose a topic for study and renewal. This particular year, we planned to study the sermons of our great teacher Roy Harrisville.

The week after July 4, Karl returned to Mule Lake, and the two of us both relaxed and worked on this book together for a few days. Then I said farewell to summer break and returned to work.

On Monday, July 15, Karl and I talked. He said that he had started vomiting in the middle of the night and didn't feel quite right. I said that I hoped to return to Mule that weekend, if he felt up to staying. Dad was down in the Twin Cities for a medical appointment but would return Wednesday.

On Tuesday night, July 16, Karl and I had our weekly Zoom call with Mike and five of our pastor friends—the same group of pastors who have spent one week together every year since 2001. This weekly call had been initiated when COVID started in 2020 as a way to cope with the shutdown. Because the call was a lifeline in the midst of chaos, we kept the call going even after COVID ended. That evening, Karl complained of nausea and said he hadn't been able to keep anything down for two days. He was drinking only Pedialyte and water. Karl was due to return to the Twin Cities the next day. His plan was to meet our dad and our sister halfway, then switch cars with Dad and return with Karen. But Karl admitted to me that he had fallen that day and was a bit lightheaded. We wrote it off to dehydration, because he could not keep anything down. We talked for about two hours and ended the call the way we do every Tuesday night, by each of us saying, "I love you" to each other. One of the other guys added to Karl, "Hey, Jake, you look like s—t." Karl laughed.

Because he did. Those are good closing words to say to each other. "I love you." Not the other words.

The next day, Karl was not responding to my texts or calls. So I called a lake neighbor, Gary, and asked him to check in on Karl. He found Karl confused and lying on the living room floor. He didn't remember falling. Again, we wrote it off to dehydration. When Karen and Dad arrived, Gary helped Karl into the car. He handed Karl two bottles of Pedialyte and told him to drink them both. Karen reported that during the ride, Karl would answer direct questions, but that he couldn't keep a conversation going. It was a long drive—Karen, Karl, two grown dogs, and a heavy, growing silence. During the last hour of the drive, Karl and his wife exchanged a few texts:

**ANGELA**
Hey, you
I'm on my way to you
I love you
Fiercely

> **KARL**
> Hey you.
> And good for you!

**ANGELA**
Madly
Deeply

> **KARL**
> Id my anything, or better
> anytime, let I, to love you how
> much I move toward you so my
> together, j kissed
> move you

Karen met Angela at the Regions Hospital ER in St. Paul. Karen dropped off both dogs at home and returned to the hospital. During the intake interview with the nurse, Karl lost consciousness. My daughter Ingrid and I joined Angela and Karen at the ER. Within an hour, a doctor said she suspected meningitis: an infection of the meninges, the protective lining around the brain and spine. This suspicion was confirmed the next day.

You can be forgiven if you read Karl's last text and thought, "Hey, he's the next e e cummings! That's some deep poetry! It was postmodern. It was deep. It was filled with double entendres! It could have multiple, valid interpretations! It was poetically, obscurely, symbolically, metaphorically awesome!"

Unfortunately, it wasn't really poetry, it was meningitis. In Karl's case, the infection and inflammation in his brain lining caused the vomiting, then the falls, then the growing confusion, and finally the poetry.

Karl was placed in a medically induced coma and intubated, and he began to fight this latest disease.

Remember Karl's words: "This book starts with cancer, but it doesn't end there." It ends with meningitis. Viral meningitis, it turns out. A rare and nasty form called varicella-zoster virus (VZV) meningitis to be precise, most likely caused by the shingles virus that Karl had as a teenager in Scotland. The chemotherapy, radiation, and bone marrow transplant that saved Karl's life also knocked back his immune system. His reduced immune system couldn't fight off the long-ago-contracted virus.

---

## ROLF (2024)

There were many positive signs and reasons for hope. The CT scans of Karl's brain and abdomen were clear. Likewise, an MRI showed no immediate signs of additional concern. Twice a day, every day, the health care workers would reduce Karl's sedation to see if he could respond and regain consciousness. At first, there was nothing. But then, on July 22, Karl showed positive signs. Angela reported that "with sedation off for the time being, he squeezed my hand countless times, opened his eyes multiple times for brief periods of time, blinked once on command, arched his eyebrows, scrunched his face, worked his jaw. All slow movements; no wild movements; he doesn't appear to be agitated or in any pain." I experienced the same positive responses. Karl squeezed my hand multiple times. I prayed out loud. When I came to Psalm 23, which I recited every time I visited him, he would react—growing a little more animated as I spoke the familiar words: "Even though I walk through the darkest valley, I fear no evil" (23:4). His eyes opened, but they could not focus.

Angela settled into "vigil mode"—creating a nest in the corner of Karl's room where she could rest and be present. All of our family and most of Karl's friends made regular visits—some from as far away as Iowa and Duluth-Superior. I was there to witness innumerable, improbable, small kindnesses done for Karl and Angela:

> My sister Karen, constantly present to translate for us with her medical expertise, to advocate for Karl with her tenacity and resolve, and to offer direct care where necessary. My sister Anne, who kindly gave Karl a

haircut and lent the steady strength that only a family firstborn can give. And her husband, Bill, and daughter Mary Ellen—as kind and bright as the sun. My ninety-three-year-old father—as strong and clear as the north wind in winter, as steady and calm as the south breeze in summer, constant in prayer, presences, and hope.

The next generation. My nieces Lucy, Nora, and Claire, who came all the way from Wilderness Canoe Base to sing and pray with Angela, to love and hug the rest of us. Karl's two elder children, TJ and Sam, working their first full-time adult jobs, while trying to navigate the turbulent rapids of a gravely ill father. My daughter Ingrid, working her own first full-time adult job, yet spending long stretches with Karl in the hospital. My son Gunnar, swinging by multiple times with a dozen or more donuts, praying for his beloved "nuncle." At times, spending the evening hours with him.

The ICU nurses—especially Isaac—so kind and patient, so caring and skilled. I recall one tech gently removing sensor probes from Karl's scalp, then carefully treating and bandaging each sore. A nurse who gently gave Karl a shave.

My wife, Amy, ever the fierce mama bear—albeit for her brother-in-law in this case—willing to take out anyone who didn't provide the absolute best for Karl (even if it was me).

Our close friends Mike, Mark, Hans, Tim, and Darrell, all of whom came by at least twice. Other friends, too: David, Dave, Greg, Ron, Tim, Mark, and so many more.

An MRI on August 5 showed that the inflammation and infection in Karl's meninges had diminished and there were promising signs of "higher function" in his brain. It also showed signs that Karl's use of his legs might be diminished or lost. His hands responded to stimuli, but his feet and lower legs did not. We worried about life for Karl in a wheelchair, with possible diminishment of mental function. Karl's health stabilized enough that the doctors made plans to transfer him to Regency Recovery Hospital in Golden Valley, Minnesota.

The annual week that Karl, Mike, and I spend each year with five other pastors at my great-grandfather's cabin Sommer Ro was set to begin on Friday, August 9. Friend David was in Florida and could not come. And Karl was in the hospital. So this year it would be only six of us. On the 9th, on our way out of town, Tim Martenson and I visited the hospital to see Karl before he was to be moved to Regency— signs were optimistic. Tim and I then drove to the cabin. Over the next two days, we were joined by four other friends.

Karl's expected move to Regency was postponed because he regressed a bit and because there wasn't yet an available bed. On Sunday evening, just as the last of the six friends were arriving at Sommer Ro, I talked by phone with my daughter Ingrid, who was at the hospital. She had just been present when some doctors delivered a tough update.

As soon as Mike arrived, he urgently asked for an update. I said, "Wait until Hans gets here. I only want to go through this once." For the next hour or two, as guys unpacked and cooked our evening meal, I wrote, edited, and rehearsed a short speech in my head. Hans finally arrived, and an impatient Mike gathered everyone onto the front porch of the cabin and said, "Okay, give it to us." I passed around a bottle of scotch—Balvenie 14, Karl's favorite—to prepare a toast. But first, I had to share the worst news.

"Guys, Karl isn't going to make it."

Mike and I both began to ugly cry. The others all cried, too. There were questions, hugs, a short speech from me, a toast. We got David on the phone and shared the news with him. We prayed. Hard. I really didn't think Karl would make it through that night.

But he did. Karl—miraculously?—fought back. He improved so much that they transferred him to Regency Recovery Hospital that Friday. Angela reported that Karl's best day was the day after he was admitted to Regency. She wrote, "Karl showed lots of movement; Nora/Lucy/Angela declared ourselves music therapists and had a 'dance party' of sorts, with rehab music provided upon request from CaringBridge folks; Karl participated 'in his own way' upon commands to move his hands/arms, which he did multiple times (think very slow drummer), later folding his hands together multiple times (free/unstrapped all day long, unlike at Regions), and even nodded when I asked up close if he wanted a kiss." Things were looking up.

---

## MIKE (2024)

"Guys, Karl isn't going to make it," Rolf choked out through his tears.

For twenty-four years, the eight of us had been gathering for a week of study, prayer, board games, pontoon cruises, golf, and lots of excellent food and drink. For each of us, those twenty-four years counted up to nearly half of our lives and more than half of our careers in ministry. Over those twenty-four years, we had collectively "gone through it all": changes in calls, almost quitting the ministry, overseas military chaplaincy deployments, divorce and remarriage, guiding parishes through the pandemic, the death of parents, a stroke, and of course, cancer diagnoses. Once upon a time, we all had young children in our households. Now all of us had begun to age into empty nesters.

"Best week of the year," Karl would often say. But this year, Karl wasn't there. He was fighting for his life back in Minnesota.

The following Sunday, August 18, 2024, Karl died.

After almost exactly a month of small, hope-filled ups and a lot of trying days of little or no changes, my best friend died. Karl's body hit a critical wall. According to the medical examiner, Karl experienced a "mucous plug causing hypoxia" (low oxygen), which led to cardiac arrest. He was resuscitated and transferred to a local hospital. Although the paramedics and doctors got his heart and lungs going again, by Sunday morning his brain activity had ceased. On Sunday afternoon, surrounded by family, life support was removed, and Karl died.

The six of us who had been at Sommer Ro had just returned from our week together. Tears and laughter (our general default toward life, suffering, and everything) had punctuated the entirety of our time together. Of course, twenty-four years of gathering in a place already full of meaning will bring back all kinds of memories and recollections. And it did: "Remember that time that Karl . . . ?" Each night we prayed and hoped that somehow, some way, Karl would rally and live. Those hopes and prayers were not answered in the way we wanted.

But Karl was right about this book: It started with cancer, but it doesn't end there. Of course, he had no idea that it would end with meningitis, caused by the chicken pox / shingles virus, which he had contracted at least forty years before.

On Saturday, August 24, we gathered at Luther Seminary's Chapel of the Incarnation, the very place where our relationships as friends, colleagues, and brothers had begun. To no one's surprise, it was a packed house. Some years ago, even before cancer, Karl had originally asked if I would preach at his funeral should he die an untimely death. Then, in 2022, when we got cancer at the same time, Karl had asked friend David to preach should he die. But David had moved to Florida. The grief I had been carrying already for two weeks, a week even before Karl had died, was so close to the surface, at times erupting in anger as well as sadness at the injustice of it all, I didn't trust myself in the least to be able to stand in a pulpit in front of God and everyone and deliver anything that sounded even remotely like the gospel, or even the English language. Fortunately, our friend Hans Wiersma, also part of the Sommer Ro crew, was tapped to preach, and I was given the privilege and responsibility of presiding at the service. "I will not be making eye contact with any of you," I told my wife and kids, who also loved Karl and Angela and their family. (Karl and Angela are the godparents of my youngest, Eleanor.) "Least of all any of you jackwagons," I added for the Sommer Ro guys.

Rolf and the bluegrass band he plays in, the Fleshpots of Egypt, would be providing a hymn sing before the service, as well as music during Communion.

The rest of the Sommer Ro gang—Darrell Kyle, Mark Tiede, Tim Martenson, and David Lillejord—were to help with serving the Lord's Supper, along with a few of Karl's former associate pastors and interns.

It's an odd thing to say—at least as odd as you might find reading this—Karl's funeral was the best funeral I've ever been a part of, and every single one of us of the Sommer Ro brotherhood have returned to and cited that day as a turning point in our grief.

Don't get me wrong. Nothing about that day changed the grim reality that—let's not beat around the bush with euphemisms like "passed" or "left us" or "was called home"—Karl was dead. As our introduction asserts, this book is written from the perspective of the "theology of the cross," a reality first lifted up by Luther in the Heidelberg Disputation in 1518, in which he says essentially, "A theologian of the cross sees something and calls it what it is."

What Rolf wrote in that introduction about suffering is that perspective of calling a thing what it is: "Suffering is ugly. Suffering scares us. Suffering shows us our own helplessness." No less so death. No less so *Karl's death*. And all that has objectively accompanied his death equally sucks. The sadness. The anger. The feelings of the injustice of it all.

Karl and I had gone through our ordeals side by side, even if separated by the necessary space for our treatments, and we were looking forward to so many things postcancer, including this book.

The truth-telling by theologians of the cross was front and center at Karl's funeral, and *that* was the turning point for our grief. Not that our grief went away. It didn't. And it hasn't to this very day. (Sometimes I wonder if it ever will.)

But, again, as we confessed in the introduction, "This book is about faithfulness as the answer to cancer—God's faithfulness, and ours." And, in the end—or perhaps as this book as a labor of love comes to an end—it turns out this book is about God's faithfulness and ours as the answer to death itself. In the face of death, we proclaim Christ crucified as God's covenant to us, the promise and the hope of God's steadfastness to us in our suffering and even in the face of death.

Everything about Karl's funeral drove us deeply into both the truth-telling of our mortality *and* the hope in the promise of the cross of Christ as God's faithfulness even in the bitter and painful aftermath of Karl's death. "I will rejoice in Jerusalem and delight in my people," we heard from the prophet Isaiah's words to his people sitting in the rubble and aftermath of their own calamity and suffering. "No more shall the sound of weeping be heard in it, or the cry of distress," even as we wept openly on that day (Isa. 65:19).

Or again from those beloved Psalms to which Karl had dedicated his life in the study and proclamation of those words: "The LORD is my light and my salvation; whom shall I fear? The LORD is the stronghold of my life; of whom shall I be afraid?" (Ps. 27:1)—words read even as we gathered in the brutal face of Karl's death and perhaps the consideration of our own.

In his sermon, Hans drove us deeply into the various aspects of Karl's death, both in the honesty of the bitterness of grief we were all experiencing and in the hope of the promise of Christ's death and resurrection: "We are here to do the gut-wrenching," he began. "Here's how this is going to go. First, I'll address any guilt that's out there"—the "coulda shoulda woulda" of second-guessing, the guilt and regret that some of us were certainly feeling in recognizing the days of symptoms Karl experienced prior to getting medical help. "Second, I'll hit the injustice of it all," Hans continued. "Third, I'll speak about Karl's life and work. Finally, I'll tell about the Crucified and Risen One, the One who died, the One who rose from the dead, the One who has swallowed up death, yes, Karl's death, in victory!" And in his proclamation, Hans didn't merely tell us *about* the gospel, the good news of God's grace and mercy even in the face of the potential gnawing guilt some may have been feeling; most importantly of all, Hans *did* the gospel to us in declaring absolution: "In the mercy of almighty God," Hans proclaimed, "Jesus Christ was given to die for you, and for his sake, God forgives you all your sins. As a called and ordained minister of the Church of Christ, and by Christ's authority, I therefore declare to you the entire forgiveness of all your sins, in the name of the Father, and of the Son, and of the Holy Spirit." Death and resurrection in answer to the emptiness of our experience of guilt and death.

But Hans reminded us that the truth-telling of Christ's cross doesn't come just through the "Talk is cheap" aspects of mere human words. "On February 15, in the year of our Lord nineteen hundred and sixty-nine, Karl was baptized into the death and resurrection of Jesus. In this way he was taken up into the life of Yeshua, the Incarnate God. Joined at the hip, as it were. . . . Our good Lord has anticipated our need, even here," Hans continued. "Christ Jesus goes beyond mere words and gives himself to us once again. And again. And again. Physically, bodily. Incarnation-style. 'This *is* my body, broken for you. This *is* my blood, shed for you, for the forgiveness of sin'" (he emphatically lingered on the word "is"). "'Give me your burden,' says the Incarnate God, 'and

163

I'll give you myself, the first fruits—the first *food*—of the new creation.'" And then Hans drove us home: "'Together,' says Christ Jesus, 'you and I will roll through this vale of tears, the valley of death. And I promise you,' says Christ, 'you will laugh again. And again. And again.' Amen."

"Thy strong word did cleave the darkness," the packed-house congregation sang in response, virtually lifting the roof off the place—one of Karl's favorite hymns. Its chorus of alleluias recalls the words that the Book of Common Prayer includes in the commendation at the end of a funeral service: "All of us go down to the dust; yet even at the grave we make our song: Alleluia, alleluia, alleluia."

Angela, of course, had keen insight in honoring Karl's requests as they had wisely had some conversation and done some planning when Karl was in the throes of his initial leukemia diagnosis. One of those requests was to have sung a song by Lyle Lovett, "Since the Last Time." The song narrates the observations of a person attending a funeral. The person being "happy" at the funeral, "seeing all those people, I ain't seen, since the last time somebody died." He recalls "everybody talking" and "telling funny stories." The story of the song concludes with a twist, a surprise Karl recognized as a key component to good comedy. (I'm not going to spoil it. Look it up and listen to it.)

When Hans and I sat with Angela to plan the service in the days before, Angela was quite insistent that this song would be featured because Karl wanted it. He wanted something "silly" at his funeral. And despite the doubts that Rolf, Hans, and I each harbored, Angela insisted on following Karl's wishes. Angela asked Rolf if his bluegrass band could do the song. "No," said Rolf, "you need a gospel band to pull off that song." The song has a swing and a "soul" to it, a gospel style that would likely put it out of reach of most. Angela was resolute. And she found a gospel pianist and singer who, along with Scott and Steve from the Fleshpots of Egypt, more than pulled it off. They positively blew the roof off the place with its big chorus: "Sing hallelujah! [Hallelujah!] Sing hallelujah! [Hallelujah!]." Rolf's dad, Del, later reported that this song is when he finally, totally lost control of his emotions.

In addition to the packed house, the amazing number of friends and seminary classmates (many of whom had traveled from far away to attend), the roof-raising hymns, and the gospel of the cross of Christ proclaimed in the face of death, I will *never* forget the performance of this song, even as we mourned, even as we rolled with Christ through this most immediate symptom of this vale of tears, even as we took into our very selves Christ's deathless presence in that bread and wine. Where I had promised prior to the service to make no eye contact with anyone, all of this steeled a courage, a hope, dare I say even a *joy* in the face of my grief. As mourning worshipers came forward with their hands and hearts open to Christ's presence, I found myself looking them right in the eye, "*This is* the body, the blood of Christ broken and shed for you."

None of this did a single, cotton-picking thing to change the immediate reality of the matter: My dearest friend, the one with whom I had traveled side by side through the ordeals of our cancer, was still dead. Even these months later, not a day goes by—not a single day—that I don't think to myself, "I should call Karl." Not a single day passes without the daily memory feature of my social media recalling some cheeky comment from Karl on a post, a photograph, a common experience. There are many days—most days, right now—when

I am ambushed by grief through something that reminds me that Karl is dead. The fact that the Minnesota Vikings are currently engaged in an amazing 2024 campaign, even as I am a Green Bay Packers fan, has been one of those weekly reminders. And it sucks.

Karl was right in so many ways about this book: It started with cancer, but it doesn't end there. It may seem to end with death. *But it doesn't even really end there.* As we lifted up in the introduction, this is a book "about life and death in the company of the God who raises the dead." This book is about faithfulness as the answer to cancer, to suffering, to broken promises, to lost opportunities, to struggling relationships, to death itself.

That faithfulness is both God's and ours. In the face of all of the symptoms of human mortality, we continue to return to the proclamation, promise, and hope of Christ's suffering, death, and resurrection as the seal of God's faithfulness to us, and indeed, to this entire planet. And we continue striving to live into our human faithfulness to each other, even in the face of all this messy mortality with which we struggle, live, and die. Through the work of the Holy Spirit first and foremost, our attempts at embodied faithfulness to each other echo in sacramental ways God's comforting faithfulness to us. In the same way the Spirit of the living Christ fills ordinary water, bread, and wine, that very same Spirit fills "ordinary *us*" too as we share one another's trials and burdens and suffering. As our pal Tim put it so eloquently one hot, summer day at Sommer Ro, "We lead brutal lives that mark us with the cross of Christ and equip us for the work of ministry."

So the Sommer Ro gang, both virtually and in person, continues to gather, sadly diminished by one, and when we gather, we actively and intentionally check in and honestly name our grief, often bluntly ripping off the bandage, hair and all: "How's your grief?" We do so in the spirit of avoiding the inevitable human repulsion to grief and suffering, in the spirit of taking Cheetos (as we've named earlier) and being intentionally present, not just in the spirit of but more importantly in the fleshiness of speaking words that matter—"I love you." And God's faithfulness spills over into our own shabby attempts. Those of us who are able still gather on Sunday afternoons to watch the Vikings with Rolf because that was part of Karl and Rolf's ritual together, and one of us isn't even a Vikings fan!

Those of us who are able still gather on Friday afternoons at a local establishment for happy hour because that was part of our liturgy together to share life, to laugh, to bear one another's burdens, and to talk smart.

Those of us who are able aim to gather monthly with Angela and the kids for Family Dinner and Game Night. None of these things are particularly "holy" in and of themselves, nor certainly are the people in and of themselves. As Karl proclaimed in his Easter Sunday sermon in 2023, when he first returned to ministry following his cancer treatment: "Let me be perfectly clear—this is not about me, or anything I've done or deserved. This is about this life-giving God of ours. This is what God does; this is who God is. Dear friends in Christ, God loves raising people from the dead."

We want to give Karl the final word. So, still quoting from that 2023 Easter sermon, here it is.[2] The last word:

> If there is one thing I've learned about the gospel in my time as a pastor, not to mention throughout my life—and if you'll bear with me, over the course of this past year my family and

I have had—if there's one thing I've learned about the gospel, it's this: God loves raising people from the dead.

*God loves raising people from the dead.* This is who God is, and what God does. Over, and over, and over again. God loves raising people from the dead.

This is what God does—literally. In the Old Testament we read that God used his prophet Elijah to raise a widow's son from the dead, restoring him to life (1 Kings 17:17–24). Jesus did the same for a widow's son in the city of Nain (Luke 7:11–17). And again, raising his friend Lazarus from the dead (John 11:1–44). And yet again, raising Jairus's daughter (Luke 8:40–56). Sons, and daughters, and friends—story after story, time and again, God raises the dead, breathing new life into forlorn flesh. This is what God does. This is who God is.

God loves raising people from the dead—literally. And so it should be no surprise that this is what the gospel promises us, in turn: that we too will be raised. This is the promise, the message that we share, that the Scriptures put to us over, and over, and over again, that we too will be raised. As the apostle Paul puts it, "If we have been united with [Christ] in a death like his, we will certainly be united with him in a resurrection like his" (Rom. 6:5).

God loves raising people from the dead. Believe it. This is the promise for us literally, but it is also the promise and the possibility for us—if you'll allow me a bit of a pretentious word—liminally; that is to say, because we will be raised from death to new life one day, . . . it is possible for us to live in newness of life on *this* day. As Paul puts it, "We [were] buried with [Christ] by baptism into death, so that, just as Christ was raised from the dead by the glory of the Father, so we too might walk in newness of life" (Rom. 6:4). The promise that we will be raised *then/someday*, means that *now /*

168

*this day*, right here and now, no matter how the powers of sin and death are at work in our lives, we can live a new life. Because God loves raising people from the dead. Now, not just on the last day, but on this day.

. . . Many of you know this intimately; you've felt it in your life, experienced it, you've seen it at work in the life of someone close to you, you've heard of it, witnessed it. And if you haven't, know that you *can*; you too can know this newness of life. I'm here to tell you that God loves raising people from the dead. From broken promises to lost opportunities to struggling relationships to looming or lingering illness. None of this can separate us from the love of God in Christ Jesus.

As I alluded to earlier, and as many of you know, my family and I have had a hard year; you've shared in it with us.

- I was diagnosed with leukemia.
- I had a bone marrow transplant, and treatments leading up to and following it. If the statistics are to be believed, I was as good as dead, and, cards on the table, I am not out of the woods, and won't be for several years; I will live for a time, now, in that shadow. But I do not fear—because God loves raising people from the dead.
- In, with, and through the faithful work of nurses and doctors and the gift of science, I have been given newness of life.
- And even if this disease should one day claim my life—even then, I will live.

And let me be perfectly clear—this is not about me, or anything I've done or deserved. This is about this life-giving God of ours.

This is what God does; this is who God is.

# EPILOGUE

## It Doesn't End There

In the introduction to this book, we recalled Karl's words, "This book starts with cancer, but it doesn't end there." We also wrote, "Karl was right. In more ways than he knew, he was right." Karl was right in several senses.

First, Karl was right in the original sense that the book is about faithfulness. Karl's idea was that although the book starts with cancer, it ends up somewhere else—namely, it ends up with the faithfulness that friends and family show to one another. With the faithfulness of what it means to suffer and survive together. And, more profoundly, with the faithfulness of God, who shows up in suffering.

Second, Karl was right in the tragic sense that the book starts with cancer and ends with meningitis. The real kick-in-the-pants aspect of Karl's death is that he had only just beat leukemia when the meningitis struck him down. It is a little spooky now to read the words Karl preached in his first sermon back from cancer on Easter Sunday 2023: "I am not out of the woods, and won't be for several years; I will live for a time, now, in that shadow." Karl knew that his leukemia might come back but also that his reduced immune system might spell the end of him. And it did.

Third, Karl was right in the *evangelical*, spiritual sense that this book ends with hope, new life, and the promise of the new creation. This book ends by bearing witness to the most profound truths of the Christian faith. The crucified Christ shows up in our suffering—even in our deaths. And the resurrected Christ walks in our midst and bears us into God's promised and preferred future. *Death will not have the last word, for the victory over death belongs to Jesus.* Following Karl's death, so many things that Karl did as a pastor and as a Christian have lived on after him. The good news that he preached to people has continued to matter in their lives. The love that Karl shared with so many throughout his life has continued to make a difference in the world. The seeds of wisdom about God, life, and the Bible that Karl shared through his ministry and writings have continued to grow and bear fruit in the lives of his congregants, students, and readers.

But most importantly, we believe that Karl's life did not end with his death because when Karl was baptized, his life was taken up into the life of the triune God. Therefore, Karl's life did not end with his death because Christ has been raised from the dead. As St. Paul writes, "If for this life only we have hoped in Christ, we are of all people most to be pitied. But in fact Christ has been raised from the dead, the first fruits of those who have died" (1 Cor. 15:19–20).

As Mike and I were putting the final touches on this manuscript, we received the tragic news that Jake, the twenty-year-old son of our friend Heather, had died unexpectedly just before Christmas. Heather had interned with Karl and played a role in Karl's funeral. Karl had at one point served her son Jake as his pastor. A short time after her son's death, Heather shared a post on social media. We include parts of her post here, with her permission:

> Another death happened today. My friend's dad died. Not by cancer, not by old age, not by overdose. Just life happened, and death is a part of life. But what is so hard about death is that it comes when you are not expecting it. Death can sneak up out of nowhere. Now, I am not a doctor, but there are some truths about death:
>
> - *Death is irreversible.* There is no medicine or surgery that can fix death.
> - *Death is universal.* Every living thing dies.
> - *Death is final.* The heart literally stops and the physical life of the body is done.

Later in her post, she added these words:

> Grief like this is hard to put into words. The stages of grief are not a box to check; they move in and around me. At times, I can laugh and remember the joy Jake brought to my life, and other times I experience the pain and freeze.

Heather concluded her post with these words:

> Being a pastor, I sometimes forget that what I preach is for me, too. Just like death is for the physical body, God's love

is the finale for our lives found in Jesus Christ. So check out these truths about God's love.

- *God's love is irreversible.* It's a love that exists within you. It cannot be reversed.
- *God's love is universal.* It's for everyone!
- *God's love is final.* It has the final word in our lives.

# FUNERAL SERMON
# *for* KARL JACOBSON

*Hans Wiersma*

*August 24, 2024 | Luther Seminary, St. Paul, MN*

Grace and peace and strength; faith and hope and love to you in the name of our Lord, Jesus Christ. Amen.

Dear Del. Dear Rolf and Karen and Anne. Dear Thursday and Sam and Lucy. Dear Nora and Claire.

Dear Angela.

Dear family and friends who have arrived at this moment to honor, to remember, to grieve, and to give thanks for our beloved Karl:

We are here to do the gut-wrenching.

---

Thank you to our friend Hans Wiersma for permission to include here the sermon he preached at Karl's funeral. It has been lightly edited for style.

Here's how this is going to go. First, I'll address any guilt that's out there. Second, I'll hit the injustice of it all. Third, I'll speak about Karl's life and work. Finally, I'll tell about the Crucified and Risen One, the One who died, the One who rose from the dead, the One who has swallowed up death, yes, Karl's death, in victory!

But I'm getting ahead of myself.

In a situation like this one, where Karl's symptoms began a day or three before he got medical help, there is second guessing—I should have done that, I failed to do this, if only I'd thought to, et cetera—there is gnawing guilt. That may take some time to get through. But I would like to hit that head-on, right here, from the pulpit:

> In the mercy of almighty God, Jesus Christ was given to die for you, and for his sake, God forgives you all your sins. As a called and ordained minister of the Church of Christ, and by Christ's authority, I therefore declare to you the entire forgiveness of all your sins, in the name of the Father, and of the Son, and of the Holy Spirit.[1]

Okay, let's move on to the next item.

It's a funny thing. Even before Karl took his last earthly breath this past Sunday, the judgments came. "It's unjust." "It's not fair." "It's wrong." Even if you knew just the most recent parts of the trajectory: Karl's cancer diagnosis two and a half years ago. The grueling treatments, the promising outcomes—at first cautious and finally, earlier this year, celebratory. And then the sudden turn, starting last month, as a deadly infection grabbed hold of Karl's body and did not let go.

Thursday, you described it so well when you compared the past two and a half years to that Disneyland ride, the Tower of Terror. You plummet down. You're jolted up. Then you jerk to a stop. Then sideways, followed by another sudden drop. Then up again. And so on. Until the ride stops and you stagger off. And we are still staggering.

"It's unjust." "It's wrong." "It's not fair." I know many of you uttered these judgments, because I heard them. I heard them uttered by Karl's friends, by members of his family, by members of my family. "It's not right," I myself said aloud and in agreement. As for me, in my mind, I immediately went to the story of Job, that biblical figure who, together with his inept friends, waxes poetic about when bad things, very bad things, happen to good people. The story of Job is, for us preacher types, a go-to when called upon to comment when unjust tragedy hits this close.

But I'm not going to go the Job route except to say these three things: (1) Job wants answers! (2) God is not happy with Job's friends, who offer crummy answers. And (3) in the end, Job gets an audience with the Almighty, hears God's long-winded answer, and is satisfied with God's answer. And to these three things, add a fourth: (4) Job's earthly life continues, *and* while he lives he never finds out why all those bad things happened to him.

Had Karl died at age eighty-four, surrounded by children and perhaps also *grandchildren*, you'd likely be making a different judgment: He had a full life, he lived to a ripe old age, and so on. Karl died about four months shy of his fifty-fifth birthday. Eighty-four years old is about how it's supposed to go. Heck, the Bible says you do well if you hit eighty. But fifty-four years old? With a wife and children? With plenty left to share with family and friends and church and community?

177

So you make a different judgment: It's not right. It's. Not. Fair.

Two years ago, Karl, together with his brother Rolf, published a book titled *Divine Laughter*, subtitled *Preaching and the Serious Business of Humor*. On page 36 of said book, there's a story about a college student offended by the unfairness embedded in one of the parables of Jesus. "This story makes me so mad," said the student. "It's not fair." Fair? Fair? And here Karl quotes a friend: "The fair's in August. It's where they judge pigs." To that we can add: "Yup, it started Thursday. You might want to avoid that part of Como Avenue for the next nine days."

Karl loved the fair; he loved living close to the fair. Until he fell ill last month, he was looking forward to the fair. "The fair's in August." That's a good quip. But right now, to those of you saying it's unfair, feeling the sting of injustice, the quip adds insult to *injury*. The injury is to your understanding of what's fair. And since God is supposed to be fair, the *injury* is also to your understanding of God. You raise your fist and defy God for explanations. Not that there's anything wrong with that. Demanding answers from God is biblical. It's part of our creaturely, defiant brokenness. If that's you, fine. God can handle it. But stick around. Stick around where the people of God gather.

For there are many others here who are, shall we say, more rehearsed with this injury, this "Why God?!" wound. In very personal ways, you've been around the block with the conundrum: If God is good, why do bad things happen to good people, even to God's people? You have learned to live with this injury. You know the injury well; you still bear the scars. But instead of shaking your fist with *fresh* anger at God, you hold back. For you know from experience there is a healing ointment, a balm, for this wound. Which is why you're here— why we're here. To hear and share that Word which makes the wounded whole. Yes, that bit is biblical too.

It's a funny thing. I've never seen someone study the Bible quite like Karl. Here's what I mean. This is what a New Testament Study Bible, Karl Edition, looks like. Upon inspection you'll see that Karl has removed the powder blue hardcover from something called the *Lutheran Study Bible*. Karl then separated the New Testament books from the rest. Next, he cut the original Bible's spine down to size. Finally (and this is my favorite part), Karl rebound this new New Testament with Star Wars–themed duct tape.

Then Karl went to work on it. Almost every page contains at least an underlined passage or a handwritten remark or question or more. If you happened to be in the same room or on the same porch as Karl, during a time of quiet repose, you'd often find Karl reading, writing, or putting sticky notes in one of his Bible concoctions. Here, for example, in the Star Wars–bound New Testament is a page filled with notes on the healing stories recorded in Mark, chapter 5. I mean, where's the original text? Yes, Karl's brand of wit, of quirk, of madcap seriousness, permeated even the Bible he used for study.

Karl leaves an impressive body of biblical and theological contributions. For you "nonprofessionals"—you normal people, that is—Karl has written many curricula, formal and informal. Especially noteworthy is his work in *Crazy Talk: A Not-So-Stuffy Dictionary of Theological Terms* and in *Crazy Book: A Not-So-Stuffy Dictionary of Biblical Terms*, as well as in *Invitation to the Psalms: A Reader's Guide for Discovery and Engagement.* And for the preacher- and Bible-teacher types, there's even more, including the aforementioned *Divine Laughter.*

By the way, my copy of *Divine Laughter* is autographed. Karl signed it, "Hans, Oh, how we needed a *Dutch Editor* for this book! In Christ, Karl." I have no idea what that means. But as many of you have learned, with Karl, insult, slander, and libel can be love languages.

But now, see, I have, against Karl's wishes, made this about Karl. Even though Karl left written instructions that he wanted his memorial service to be about God. So, I'll end this part with an admonishment: Do you have Karl memories and Karl stories? Based on what I heard at a couple of informal gatherings yesterday, I know the answer is an enthusiastic *yes.* So keep telling those stories, share them, for when you do, it's more than likely that laughter will ensue. For as it is written (in *Divine Laughter,* page 96): "The ability to laugh in the midst of life's pain is a subversive witness to hope. . . . In short, the ability to express joy in sorrow, laughter in the midst of tears, is a witness to purpose and meaning when so much seems purposeless and meaningless." Laughter, in other words, is good for the soul.

It's a funny thing. This incarnation. This oft-told story, this breakthrough narrative, about the almighty Creator of heaven and earth being shoehorned into human history, shoehorned into a human body, born of a woman, raised in a land and in a religion in a faraway corner of a brutal empire. I mean, c'mon. You can imagine how an early hearer responded to the story, laughing in disbelief.

"You mean to tell us the Creator of the universe took on flesh like ours and lived a life like ours? And then when he got some notice, some renown, he got into trouble with the powers that be? And instead of overwhelming those powers, he succumbed to them? He was arrested, mocked, beaten, tried, executed, and buried?! That's funny. Twisted. But funny."

"Well," says our storyteller from long ago, "that's not the end of it."

"There's more?" asks the incredulous hearer.

"Yeah," says the teller. "Some women came to the tomb to give him a proper burial. They brought some good-smelling oils to mask the smell of death. But when they arrived, the tomb was empty. Then the dead man started appearing alive—appearing and disappearing to his followers."

Hearer: "Wait. What?"

Teller: "Yup."

Hearer: "Does this Incarnate Deity have a name?"

Teller: "Yeshua. That's Hebrew for 'God *Is* Salvation.'"

Hearer: "Really? 'God Is Salvation'? Isn't that kind of obvious?"

Teller: "I suppose."

Hearer: "And you say he was executed on a Roman cross?"

Teller: "That's right."

Hearer: "A bit gruesome, don't you think?"

Teller: "Hey, I'm just the messenger."

Hearer: "Hmm. Interesting. You got my attention. What else is there?"

Teller: "Well. Listen up . . ."

———

Many of you know this story of God's incarnation well. Very well. Some of you, like Karl, have even been called to devote your life to learning and teaching about the incarnation—its breadth and depth, its original context of first-century Jews living in Roman-occupied Judea—to telling and shaping the message for current contexts and modern hearers.

Our beloved Karl is just one of many, many, many regular people over the centuries who hear the call. Not only the call to trust and follow the Crucified One. But also the call to learn the Scriptures, to plumb them, to discern them. To understand better than most how the Scripture reveals the life of God through Jesus Christ. And finally to proclaim the revelation to others. To tell the funny, life-saving story. In all its many dimensions.

Okay, home stretch here.

On February 15, in the year of our Lord nineteen hundred and sixty-nine, Karl was baptized into the death and resurrection of Jesus. In this way he was taken up into the life of Yeshua, the incarnate God. Joined at the hip, as it were.

Now fast-forward fifty-four and a half years to the present. Karl lived his life submerged in those waters for fifty-four and a half years. And Angela, you showed up on that timeline at some point while the both of you were college students. And then ten years ago, you showed up on Karl's timeline for keeps. The two of you built your life together on the promises of God Incarnate. Promises that include the communion of saints, the forgiveness of sins, the resurrection of your bodies, and the new life without end.

Speaking of the forgiveness of sin, the other day you said, "You know, Karl's not perfect." I thought, Uh oh, here it comes. "It was his job to finish the taxes," you explained, pointing to the dining room table. "And there they are, still not done." That's the kind of forgiveness of sins the life of Jesus inspires!

But here's another promise straight from the mouth of your Lord. This one's not in the Creed, though. Too bad, really. Because, right now, this promise is especially for you. And Del, you too. All of you. This promise is for all of you, of course. Because the untimely, unfair death of a spouse, a son, a dad, a brother, a close relative, a dear friend is a heavy, heavy burden. We are not built to bear such a burden alone. And so Christ says to you, to all of you:

> Come to me, all you who are weary and are carrying heavy burdens, and I will give you rest. Take my yoke upon you, and learn from me, for I am gentle and humble in heart, and you will find rest for your souls. For my yoke is easy, and my burden is light. (Matt. 11:28–30 NRSVue)

Easier said than done, you say? How am I to muster up so much willpower to just hand over my burden like that? Why doesn't God just take away the burden, the grief, altogether? Snap of the fingers and—poof—it's gone? But that's not how this life works. It's exactly *because* you love so much that your heart breaks open.

And yet our good Lord has anticipated our need, even here. Christ Jesus goes beyond mere words and gives himself to us once again. And again. And again. Physically, bodily. Incarnation-style. "This *is* my body, broken for you. This *is* my blood, shed for you, for the forgiveness of sin." "Give me your burden," says the incarnate God, "and I'll give you myself, the first fruits—the first *food*—of the new creation." "Together," says Christ Jesus, "you and I will roll through this vale of tears, the valley of death. And I promise you," says Christ, "you will laugh again. And again. And again."

Amen.

# NOTES

## Chapter 1 Diagnosis

1. The concept is found throughout Luther's writings. For example, see "Confession Concerning Christ's Supper (1528)," in *Word and Sacrament III*, ed. Robert H. Fischer, Luther's Works 37 (Fortress, 1961), 306.

2. These include Psalms 16, 27, 46, 121, and more.

3. Malcolm Gladwell, *The Tipping Point: How Little Things Make a Big Difference* (Little, Brown, 2000); see 163–66.

4. Large Catechism, in *Book of Concord*, trans. and ed. Theodore G. Tappert (Muhlenberg, 1959), 365.

5. "Jerry Seinfeld: The Uncomfortable Feeling of Awkward Humor Is Okay," *The Free Press*, May 12, 2024, https://www.thefp.com/p/jerry-seinfeld-duke-commencement.

## Chapter 2 Treatment

1. A favorite story about Karl when he was eleven years old: Rolf and their parents were at Mayo for surgery, so a neighbor, Keith Homstad, was asked to look after Karl after school. During school, some kid said to Karl, "How's your peg-leg brother?" So Karl—who was never the best at math—smashed him in the nose with his math textbook. He was sent to the principal's office, and Keith Homstad was called in. The principal sent Karl home with Keith, along with a stern admonition to tell our parents what Karl had done. In the car, Keith said, "You shouldn't have done this, Karl. And I would have done the same thing. We'll keep this between us. Your parents will never know about this." And they didn't . . . until Karl told them the story years later. Good for Keith. And Karl.

2. By the way, Rolf's favorite oncologist, who goes by the name of Dr. Sarcoma (not really, but that is what Rolf calls him), told Rolf that nothing Rolf did or did not do contributed to his contracting sarcoma. Sarcoma is not a lifestyle-dependent disease. It isn't caused by smoking, diet, favorite football team, or which band instrument you play.

3. Martin Luther, *Lectures on Galatians 1535: Chapters 1–4*, ed. Jaroslav Pelikan, Luther's Works 26 (Concordia, 1962), 30. Emphasis added.

4. See also Psalms 4:1; 13:3; 27:7; 55:2; 86:1; 102:2; 108:6; 119:145; 143:1, 7.

5. Eugene Peterson, *Working the Angles: The Shape of Pastoral Integrity* (Eerdmans, 1987), 45.

6. Peterson, *Working the Angles*, 47.

7. Peterson, *Working the Angles*, 44.

## Chapter 3  Meals and Milestones

1. Tony Campolo, *The Kingdom of God Is a Party* (Word, 1990), 28.

2. Kate Bowler, *Everything Happens for a Reason: And Other Lies I Have Loved* (Random House, 2018).

3. Kate Bowler, "Death, the Prosperity Gospel, and Me," Opinion, *The New York Times*, February 13, 2016, https://www.nytimes.com/2016/02/14/opinion/sunday/death-the-prosperity-gospel-and-me.html.

4. The quotation comes from Nietzsche's work *Götzen-Dämmerung*, which appeared in English as *The Twilight of the Idols*.

5. This adage has been attributed to many sources. The oldest attestation we can find is from the February 26, 1959, edition of the *Amarillo Globe-Times*, which reported that at a PTA meeting, a man named Charles Eads "claimed the teacher's job is to take 25 or 30 live wires and make sure they are well grounded. Then he made a statement that might give pause to a student of psychology. It's worded peculiarly. The statement is, 'Hurt people hurt people.'" "Quote Origin: Hurt People Hurt People," Quote Investigator, September 15, 2019, https://quoteinvestigator.com/2019/09/15/hurt/.

6. Judith Guest, *Ordinary People* (Viking, 1976).

## Chapter 4  Laughter

1. *Comedians in Cars Getting Coffee*, season 4, episode 3, "Opera Pimp," directed and produced by Jerry Seinfeld, featuring Robert Klein, aired July 3, 2014, on Crackle.

2. Stephen Prothero, *Religious Literacy: What Every American Needs to Know—and Doesn't* (HarperCollins, 2007), 27–29.

3. Here are the answers, in case you don't know. The four Gospels: John, Paul, George, and Ringo. Okay, not really. They are Matthew, Mark, Luke, and John. The first five books of the Bible (the Torah or Pentateuch) are Genesis, Exodus, Leviticus, Numbers, and Deuteronomy. And the first amendment of the US Constitution says, "Congress may make no law respecting an establishment of religion or prohibiting its free exercise." PS: George Will was often heard to quip that "Congress may make no law" are the five best words in the English language.

4. Quotes from CaringBridge entries have been lightly edited for style.

5. "Jerry Seinfeld: The Uncomfortable Feeling of Awkward Humor Is Okay," *The Free Press*, May 12, 2024, https://www.thefp.com/p/jerry-seinfeld-duke-commencement. Emphasis added.

## Chapter 5  Survival

1. *Lutheran Book of Worship* (Augsburg, 1978), p. 131.

2. *Lutheran Book of Worship*, p. 131.

3. Richard W. Nysse, "Commentary on Daniel 3:1–30," Working Preacher, accessed April 25, 2025, https://www.workingpreacher.org/commentaries/narrative-lectionary/daniel/commentary-on-daniel-31-30.

4. Want more church crazy talk? You're in luck! See Rolf A. Jacobson, ed., *Crazy Talk: A Not-So-Stuffy Dictionary of Theological Terms*, rev. ed. (Augsburg, 2017). And also, Rolf A. Jacobson, Karl N. Jacobson, and Hans H. Wiersma, eds., *Crazy Book: A Not-So-Stuffy Dictionary of Biblical Terms*, rev. ed. (Augsburg Books, 2019). They're pretty funny.

5. "The Light of Love Comes Shining Through," by Steve Thompson, copyright 2005. Used by permission.

## Chapter 6  Death

1. J. R. R. Tolkien, *The Fellowship of the Ring*, 2nd ed. (Houghton Mifflin, 1965), 41.

2. Karl's sermon has been lightly edited for style.

## Appendix  Funeral Sermon for Karl Jacobson

1. This version of the absolution is Wiersma's slight editing and combining of two options of the absolution from the *Lutheran Book of Worship* (Augsburg Books, 1978), 78.

# DISCUSSION QUESTIONS

*Note:* These questions are offered as a way of enlivening the content and theology of this book, as well as the authors' personal memories, experiences, and suffering, such that the book might provide insight to your own (or your small group's) memories, experiences, or suffering. Accordingly, the questions are offered in what is hopefully an intentional and consistent pattern:

1. *Personal*—These questions will invite you into some reflection on your own personal experiences and encounters with cancer perhaps, but also with any sort of sudden and disorienting diagnosis or life event. As Karl asserts in the introduction, "This book isn't about cancer . . . but it starts there" (p. xii).
2. *Scriptural*—These questions will invite you to grapple with the Bible, mostly through the Scripture passages offered and cited in the book itself. There will be a

few encouragements and invitations to go deeper or further into a particular Scripture passage or theme. (For example, see question 2 in chapter 4 and its invitation to review or familiarize yourself with the Gospels' accounts of Jesus's resurrection.) However, our intent is that these questions neither assume expertise on your part nor require some biblical expertise; nor should they make you feel dumb about what you "should or shouldn't know" concerning the Bible. Rather, we hope that you, along with us, hear and trust anew the promise and grace of God in Christ Jesus that the Word delivers.

3. *Responsive*—These questions will invite you to think about and respond to a person in your life who has or is experiencing the disorientation and shock of bad news through a diagnosis or any of the countless other ways human beings suffer. In short, these questions might help you both imagine and act in going to those who suffer, to take Cheetos, and to say, "I love you." The responsiveness of medical teams, family, and friends, of which the authors have only been grateful recipients, is a key component to their experiences of suffering, treatment, recovery, and death. It is our hope that perhaps these questions might elicit a similar response as that of Jesus to the legal expert whose questions inspire the parable of the good Samaritan: "Go and do likewise" (Luke 10:25–37). Not in theoretical abstractions and thoughts, but in embodied realities of grace, mercy, and love for those who suffer.

## Chapter 1  Diagnosis: Dealing with the Disorienting News of Cancer

1. The authors suggest that their encounters with a sudden and disorienting cancer diagnosis are not unlike "any significant, sudden trauma: a heart attack, the sudden death of a loved one, a major accident, the unexpected loss of a job, being the victim of a crime, and so on" (p. 17).

   ▪ Reflect on a time that you have experienced such trauma, either in your own life or in the lives of your loved ones.

   ▪ What are some of the specifics you remember about that moment of receiving that news? How did you absorb it?

2. At the outset of this chapter, we note that Psalm 30:7 declares, "Then you [LORD] hid your face; I was terrified"—a theme or feeling of fear and abandonment by God expressed numerous times in various ways throughout the Bible. Reflecting on his ordeal in the belly of the great fish, for example, the prophet

Jonah observes, "You hurled me into the depths, into the very heart of the seas" (Jon. 2:3 NIV), this after also being preserved and vomited out. From his cross, Jesus questions God's presence and expresses his own feelings of abandonment (Jesus does this!): "My God, my God, why have you forsaken me?" (Mark 15:34 NIV).

- How do these expressions of perceived abandonment—which are part of the Bible itself—strike you?

- Thinking about your own encounters with the shock and disorientation of diagnosis (or experiences like diagnosis), how did you express this to or about God?

- Even with these expressions of abandonment, the witness of Scripture is that of God's faithfulness. Rolf describes that faithfulness as experienced through people (p. 5). Mike uses the sacramental language of encounters with God's faithfulness "in, with, and under" suffering (p. 11). Karl reflects on

Psalm 23 as a lens through which to see God's faith-fulness (p. 16). How have you experienced, seen, or been sustained in suffering by God's faithfulness?

3. Who do you know who is grappling with the dis-orientation and shock of bad news? In what spe-cific way(s) might you be their experience of God's faithfulness?

## Chapter 2  Treatment: When God Shows Up in Your Suffering

1. Rolf remembers a story about a woman who, shortly after his diagnosis, sought to make sense of the situa-tion or find a logical reason for it: "If you [addressing Rolf's mother, Katherine] had served your family a diet full of fresh fruits and vegetables, Rolf wouldn't have cancer" (p. 42).

   Reflecting on a previous tragedy in his life, Karl shares what his father had said in response: "God is in it." Karl goes on to explain that "Dad didn't mean,

'This is God's plan,' or 'God has a reason,' but instead that I could expect that this God of ours . . . shows up when the walls of the valley of the shadow of death are closing in" (p. 44).

Mike names some specific ways he believes God showed up during his suffering: "in the cancer veterans in my life and their wealth of experience, . . . in the presence of my friends and our shared sense of humor, . . . in the knowledge, expertise, and skill of my doctors, . . . [in] the presence of my wife Kari and our kids" (pp. 40–41).

- Have you ever had the experience of someone trying to say something helpful (or, at the very least, reasonable) that came out sideways and was unhelpful?

- What did that person say? What do you think their good intention was (assuming they weren't a total schmuck)? What was not helpful about their assertion?

- Reflect on a time when you might say "God showed up" in the midst of suffering.

2. At the beginning of this chapter, Psalm 130:1–2a, 5–6 gives voice to some deeply human words, emotions, and experiences that well up "out of the depths" (v. 1).
   - Can you identify some of those words, emotions, and experiences named in that psalm?

   - Throughout this chapter, a number of psalms are lifted up as examples of both God's silence and God's anticipated response in the face of that apparent silence: Psalms 109:1, 28; 35:22–23 (p. 34); 32:3–4 (pp. 35–36); and 69:13–18 (p. 48). Karl cites Jesus's prayer in the garden and his cry from the cross as examples of speaking "to God's silence" (p. 34), and he also cites "a vulnerable child born to a virgin in a cattle stall and placed in the animals' feeding trough" as well as "an innocent man nailed to a cross and left to die" (p. 46) as examples of God showing up in life's lowest lows. Are there other

195

stories you can think of from the Bible where someone speaks to God's silence or their perception of hopelessness in their predicament?

3. Beginning on page 33, Karl reflects on three aspects of silence: (1) relational silence, (2) God's silence, and (3) his own silence.

   ▪ For whom might you fill the void of relational silence and in what specific way(s)?

   ▪ Echoing question 3 from the previous chapter (i.e., Who do you know who is grappling with the disorientation and shock of bad news? In what specific way(s) might you be their experience of God's faithfulness?), how might your attempts to fill relational silence also be God's response in the midst of experiencing seemingly apparent silence from God?

- Have you ever found yourself praying for others "to get out of [y]our own head, out of [y]our own way, and trust that others are praying for [you] too" (p. 35)?

## Chapter 3 Meals and Milestones: How We Show Up for Each Other

1. Rolf describes a meal with his father's friend Jerry (beginning on p. 53), a meal he links to Jesus's words from John 10 about abundant life (pp. 55–56); Isaiah's vision of a mountaintop feast (pp. 56–57); a joy-filled feast of abundance from Deuteronomy (p. 57); and the prepared table in the presence of one's enemies from Psalm 23 (p. 59). Reflect on a time when you experienced a similar scenario in your life.

2. Reflect on the imagery of those pieces of Scripture above, of abundance, joy, and honor. Are there other stories from the Bible you can think of in which abundance, joy, and/or honor are brought to life through food or a meal?

3. Throughout this book and its questions, you have been encouraged to think of someone in your life who might be experiencing significant challenges. There are some dos and don'ts that are suggested in this chapter. As you continue to think about this person (or persons), review these dos and don'ts. Jot down some notes about how these suggestions might apply to you and your relationship with this person. If you are gathering with a group around this book, share your thoughts with others.

   - *"Do not* provide easy answers—or really any answers—for why something is happening to a good person" (p. 64). What are some of the "easy answers" lifted up in this section?
   - Do "admit to yourself that you may not want to go. . . . Go anyway" (p. 72). Why might you—or any human being—not want to go?

- Do "bring Cheetos" (p. 73). What would "Cheetos" be in the context of the person about whom you have been thinking?
- Do "say, 'I love you'" (p. 83).
- Do "stick with it" (p. 83).
- "Do not be too hard on yourself" (p. 84).

**Chapter 4  Laughter: Finding Joy in the Midst of Illness and Disability**

1. When have you experienced humor in the midst of something otherwise categorically unfunny?

2. What do you note about the authors' reflections on laughter and joy as spiritual gifts, as "ways of receiving God's Easter promise" (p. 91)? What are some

elements of the Easter story about which we might find God getting the last laugh? (By the way, you can find the Easter accounts in the Gospels of Matthew [chap. 28], Mark [chap. 16], Luke [chap. 24], and John [chaps. 20 and 21], and you can find Peter's and Paul's reflections on the resurrection in Acts 2:14–47, 1 Corinthians 15, and 2 Corinthians 4 and 5 as well.)

3. As you continue to think about the person who suffers in your life, are there particular observations about humor and laughter offered by the authors you find to be helpful? Challenging? How might the authors' thoughts about humor and laughter equip you for your relationship with this person who suffers in particularly unfunny ways?

## Chapter 5 Survival: Living in the Aftermath of Illness

1. Back in chapter 1, you were invited to remember an incident—a diagnosis, a heart attack, the sudden death of a loved one, a major accident, the unexpected loss of a job, being the victim of a crime, and so on.

Discussion Questions

- Discuss what you remember about the eventual aftermath: coming to grips with a new normal, recovery or picking up the pieces, the upset and turmoil that had to be dealt with.

- What are some of the specifics you remember? Were there uncertainties you had to face? How were others around you affected by this new normal? Can you remember any aspects of trying to maintain old normalcies and routines in the new normal?

2. Three of the pieces of Scripture cited in this chapter—Psalm 30:1–3 (p. 111), 1 Corinthians 15:52–57 (pp. 114–15), and Psalm 144:1–2 (pp. 118–19)—use the metaphorical imagery of a battle and the hope for victory.
   - What in these words and their imagery do you find helpful? What do you find challenging?

201

- On pages 120–23, Karl reflects on the story of Shadrach, Meshach, and Abednego from Daniel 3. It is often important to note both who is the subject of the action and who is the beneficiary. How would you give voice to this both in this story and in the readings above?

3. Throughout these questions, you have been encouraged to think about a person with whom you share life who has gone through or who is going through a diagnosis or trauma. Exploring what you have in this chapter in grappling with aftermaths, are there thoughts you have about your ongoing relationship with this person? (Perhaps it might help to review the dos and don'ts from chap. 3.)

## Chapter 6 Death: Recurrence, Fear, Exhaustion, and Hope

1. What are you afraid of?

2. The authors note the role and lessons of the psalms of trust in confronting fears, citing Psalms 23:4a, 27:3, and 46:1–3 (p. 140). Inserting the fear (or fears) you name above, can you rephrase those psalms in the terms of your fears?

3. On pages 161 and following, Mike reflects on the truth-telling that comes with being a theologian of the cross: "A theologian of the cross sees something and calls it what it is" (p. 161).

   - Review the notes you might have jotted down throughout this study. What have been some of the truths you have spoken about diagnosis, treatment, suffering, and/or death?

- What have been some of the truths you have spoken about God in the midst of these things?

- On pages 166 and following, Mike names some regular aspects of the Sommer Ro gang's life together that have continued to reflect God's promised faithfulness through their faithfulness to each other, even without Karl: Sunday afternoons together to watch Vikings games, Friday afternoon happy hours, family dinners. What thoughts and desired actions come to mind for you as you think about your life together with those who suffer? With those who no longer suffer but are dead?